when you're not
expecting

when you're not expecting

An Infertility Survival Guide

Calm Your Emotions
Strengthen Your Relationships
Recover from Pregnancy Loss
Re-balance Your Life
Access Helpful Resources

Constance Hoenk Shapiro, M.S.W., Ph.D.

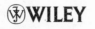

WILEY

John Wiley & Sons Canada, Ltd.

Library and Archives Canada Cataloguing in Publication Data

Shapiro, Constance Hoenk
   When you're not expecting : an infertility survival guide /
Constance Hoenk Shapiro.

Includes index.
ISBN 978-0-470-73641-8

   1. Infertility.   2. Infertility—Psychological aspects.   I. Title.

RC889.S49 2010   618.1'78   C2009-905174-5

Production Credits
Cover and interior design: Pat Loi
Typesetting: Thomson Digital
Cover photo: iStockphoto.com
Printer: Friesens

John Wiley & Sons Canada, Ltd.
6045 Freemont Blvd.
Mississauga, Ontario
L5R 4J3

Printed in Canada

1 2 3 4 5 FP 14 13 12 11 10

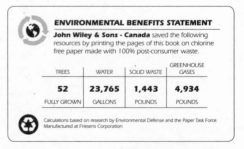

ENVIRONMENTAL BENEFITS STATEMENT
John Wiley & Sons - Canada saved the following resources by printing the pages of this book on chlorine free paper made with 100% post-consumer waste.

TREES	WATER	SOLID WASTE	GREENHOUSE GASES
52	**23,765**	**1,443**	**4,934**
FULLY GROWN	GALLONS	POUNDS	POUNDS

Calculations based on research by Environmental Defense and the Paper Task Force. Manufactured at Friesens Corporation

Contents

Contents

Acknowledgments

I owe gratitude to so many people who have confided in me, supported me, and contributed to this book.

To my family and loved ones: my husband Stuart Shapiro, my son Daniel Shapiro, Kit Transue, and Kara Otterness, who patiently encouraged me as I juggled the joys of motherhood with offering therapy, conducting academic research, and organizing infertility conferences. I offer special gratitude to my daughter Adrienne Shapiro, whose medical expertise provided incisive input to each chapter.

To my former and current students: Margaret Bane St. Peters, Frances Siegel, Emily Lombardo, and Diana Parry, who provided timely research, proofreading, and social networking efforts.

To my dear friends: Ellen deLara and Ellen Jacobsen, whose unflagging professional expertise and suggestions offered new perspectives for me to include.

Acknowledgments

To administrators and colleagues at the University of Illinois, whose support ranged from providing me with a sabbatical semester that I used to write many chapters to providing nitty-gritty assistance with technology issues, with which Andrea Fierro and Diane Wolfe Marlin were particularly helpful.

To my colleagues at John Wiley and Sons, Canada, who not only believed in this book but also provided the editing input that helped make the book so much better.

To my clients, without whose words this book could never have come into being!

Introduction

When I embarked on my own infertility journey many years ago, I felt completely lost. I had no map to suggest the pathways that might lie ahead. I knew no infertile women — or at least not any who talked openly about their difficulties getting pregnant or their pregnancy losses. My gynecologist was willing to do some preliminary tests on me, but he never once suggested that I seek help at an infertility clinic. And when I said to my husband and family that I was feeling emotionally under siege, no one knew how to comfort me. Even worse, I couldn't figure out how to solve this problem — after all, hadn't I spent years trying *not* to become pregnant? Now that I was ready to be a mother, why wouldn't my body cooperate? For several years my husband and I endured tests and treatments, and still my period appeared like clockwork. I, who once had believed that trying hard was the best path to success, was stymied. Didn't anyone understand how desperate I was to have a baby?

Sound familiar? Although my personal scenario may not mirror every detail of your unique quest for motherhood, I suspect you can identify with the loneliness, the frustration, and the sadness. These are challenging feelings, and no one can appreciate them as well as another woman struggling to conceive and have a healthy pregnancy.

Infertility is a journey that is unique for each person, yet it has some well-traveled pathways. Some experiences will be familiar to almost everyone who is infertile. Others will differ if you have pregnancy losses or IVF failures, if you are single, if you are in a lesbian relationship, or if you are already a birth mother and are trying to conceive again. The chapters ahead discuss all these twists in the road.

The survival strategies in this book come from over 200 women and couples I have known and listened to in my 20 years as an infertility counselor. They represent a sisterhood of survivors, eager to share their emotions, coping strategies, and ultimate triumphs. I have disguised identifying information to protect their confidentiality, but I have retained their wisdom and creativity. Of course, my life too has been shaped by infertility, and you will hear my voice in the therapeutic tips at the end of each chapter, as well as intermingled with the voices of the women whose experiences mirror yours.

A major purpose of this book is to introduce you to these traveling companions who made choices about their infertility that allowed them to gain more control over their lives. You will encounter a variety of spirited and sympathetic women who openly share the wisdom they have acquired. Whatever your current situation, you will find stories that reflect and respond to issues you are dealing with right now. And beyond the empathy extended by the voices in this book, you will also find the practical strategies these women used to take back their lives that had been hijacked by infertility.

About half of all infertility is due to male factors, as many of you reading this book are well aware. If you have a male partner, regardless of who is receiving treatment, *both* of you are feeling a wealth of emotions associated with your collective hope of getting pregnant. However, women and men experience infertility differently. Both feel the apprehension that they cannot easily have children, but women often feel on the outside of what I think of as "The Club." Surrounded by pregnant and parenting peers, infertile women feel awkward and often angry as they are expected to take joy in others' baby showers, birth announcements, christenings, holiday celebrations, and birthdays. Gradually a woman may begin to feel that everyone but her is either pregnant or pushing a stroller. And whether pregnant friends babble on about Lamaze classes or are awkwardly silent in an effort to respect a friend's pain, women's day-to-day lives, as opposed to the lives of men, are intrinsically more tied to conceiving, pregnancy, birth, and nursing, the absence of which can cause a visceral sense of loss. I encourage you to share this book with the men in your life — partners, brothers, fathers, and friends. Men often struggle to understand infertility as women experience it. However, once they have this understanding, men can be very open to suggestions for how they can offer support, and they may need encouragement from you before they can ask for emotional comfort for themselves. Infertility is a challenge to the *couple*, and it will shape your relationship in unexpected ways. So this book includes the voices of men. You will hear their stories and suggestions about ways to communicate with them more clearly.

An increasing number of lesbians and single women are confronting social biases and declaring their wish to have a birth child. Some may have children from previous relationships, and some may never have been pregnant. Many have close and supportive networks of friends and family. But *social factor infertility*, or the lack of a male partner, propels many lesbians and single women to seek the services of infertility specialists and adoption agencies. Although their issues often are not that different from married heterosexual couples who desperately want to become pregnant, lesbians and single women face unique challenges on the pathway to parenthood. This book discusses those challenges, with a range of voices offering creative strategies as well as empathy and understanding.

My own personal anguish during my years of infertility made me vow that if I ever had a baby I would continue to stay connected to the infertile sisterhood with whom I felt such shared experience. I was ultimately fortunate to have two children, but parenthood did not erase the powerful memories of my own infertility. I plunged back into my work as a clinical social worker, devoting my counseling exclusively to infertile couples and individuals. I was amazed that people came from many miles to share their anguish and frustrations, as well as their courage and triumphs. The years progressed, and I found that I was learning more from my clients than my own experience ever taught me. As I spoke with others about the challenges of their infertility, I found myself offering ideas and perspectives that I had picked up from my ever-widening network of infertile acquaintances. And I found my respect growing for the determination and creative solutions demonstrated by my clients and their own infertile friends.

Ultimately, I came to realize that the women who had shared their journeys with me had exactly what every woman struggling with infertility needs, and what you will find as you read on: a wealth of maps, a generous supply of strategies, and an abundance of wisdom to share.

One

Infertility:
The Journey Begins

The reasons for deciding to try to become pregnant are
different for each woman, as you will notice when you think
about your own reasons. Perhaps you were surrounded by pregnant women and new parents, and the time felt right; perhaps
your education or your financial circumstances were at a place
where you were ready to take on parenthood as a new life
challenge; perhaps your parents, your siblings, or your in-laws
increasingly asked when you were going to add a new member
to the family; or, even more likely, perhaps you and your partner began to look at your life together and think about what
becoming parents would mean. So, after weeks or months of
sharing doubt and anticipation, you found yourself perched
hopefully on the brink of a new life stage: parenthood.

But if you are reading this book, the brink may be feeling
more like a precipice. Your hopes of becoming a mother have
not been realized. You are filled with apprehension about why
it is taking so long to achieve something that seems effortless for

everyone else. Your questions about where to go from here have sent you to the bookstore, the Internet, and your gynecologist, and the word *infertility* is becoming all too familiar. This is not a journey you want to embark on, but you realize the best next step is to face this challenge.

Perhaps you can identify with some of the following scenarios:

"Bob and I had stopped using birth control, and after about a year I began to feel worried about not becoming pregnant. Since we are in our twenties, my doctor gave me some charts and told me to keep trying — he didn't seem concerned. But it's been 18 months now, and I'm beginning to think that the word *infertility* may apply to me."

"As a lesbian I have always known that becoming pregnant would present its own set of challenges. My partner and I have not been able to find a physician in our small community who is willing to work with us, so we're resigned to seeking help in a city that is a three-hour drive away."

"My mother took DES when she was pregnant with me, so I have always known that pregnancy might not be as easy for me as it is for others. When John and I were engaged, I told him that he deserved to know about the medical problems associated with DES, so my gynecologist talked with both of us and gave us some literature. John said he loved me and that we would face this together. Now that we've been trying to get pregnant for over a year, I'm really worried that this will be a big struggle."

"I was able to become pregnant for the first time with no problem. We have an adorable four-year-old daughter. But we've been trying to get pregnant for the past two years and now our doctor has referred us to an infertility clinic, because she can't figure out what the problem is."

"After two years of being unable to conceive, Jack was referred by my gynecologist to a urologist, while I underwent some preliminary procedures. My test results all came back as normal, but when Jack's semen analysis results came back, we were both floored to learn that his sperm count is low and the quality of his sperm is poor. When the urologist talked with us about artificial insemination by donor, we felt the bottom fall out of our lives."

Whether infertility creeps more persistently into your worries about why you are not becoming pregnant, or whether you have an inkling of the difficulties you might experience with getting pregnant, it is still a rude awakening to realize that pregnancy will not come easily. As the rude awakening becomes a diagnosis of infertility, women and their partners begin to grapple with the meaning of this diagnosis, in terms of both the medical interventions and the uncertainty now associated with dreams of parenthood.

Infertility Testing

Most couples are apprehensive but eager to establish the source of their infertility as quickly as possible. The statistics regarding who is physically responsible for infertility are split roughly down the middle between men and women (about 40 percent each). In a surprising 20 percent of cases, both the man and the woman have physical issues or the source of the problem is unknown. With that in mind, it is important to be prepared for the reality that some couples cannot get the definitive answers they seek, even after a comprehensive diagnostic workup. Knowing this ahead of time will prepare you for what is likely to be an ongoing series of tests. Ultimately, a small percentage of couples may never know the source of the problem.

You and your partner will feel more comfortable beginning your diagnostic workup if you have some idea of what to expect. Understanding the importance of these initial tests will enable you to choose doctors who perform these procedures on a regular basis. After all, an appropriate diagnostic workup is the foundation on which to develop a successful treatment plan. So without going into too much medical detail or jargon, here I discuss some of the conditions that can contribute to a couple's infertility and the procedures that are typically used to identify these conditions.

Infertility in women is often caused by a problem in ovulation or an anatomical problem, such as blocked or damaged fallopian tubes. In men, fertility may be affected by sperm quantity or quality. It is important to evaluate both partners for conditions that are contributing to their infertility. Typically women are tested before their male partners, but there is no reason for this, especially if you are trying to proceed as efficiently as possible. Basic testing of both you and your partner could be completed in six to eight weeks.

A urologist, preferably one who specializes in male infertility, will typically start with a comprehensive medical history and physical examination, which may include blood work, ultrasound testing, genetic testing, or specialized tests on the semen. A semen analysis, the foundation for male fertility evaluation, should include semen volume, sperm count, *motility* (speed), and *morphology* (shape). This test can reveal the most common male infertility factors: *azoospermia* (no sperm cells are being produced) and *oligospermia* (few sperm cells are produced).

Sometimes sperm cells are malformed or die before they can reach the egg. Because of the variation that can occur in semen samples, most doctors will request two separate specimens at least two weeks apart. Do not expect your partner to be thrilled at this, but do express to him how vital his participation is in the diagnostic workup. Additional testing may be done to measure male hormone levels, since a hormonal deficiency can easily be treated and result in restoring normal fertility.

While your male partner is being evaluated, you should pursue an infertility workup as well. Many of the appropriate tests can be performed by an ob-gyn. Often, however, a *reproductive endocrinologist*, a physician who specializes in infertility and hormonal problems, can evaluate your needs more quickly. After an initial history and physical examination, an evaluation of ovarian function is accomplished by examining you at the beginning of your cycle, at the time of presumed ovulation, and again approximately one week later. Pelvic ultrasound studies and serum hormone analysis provide the physician with a picture of whether or not ovulation is occurring properly. *Ovarian reserve* (the potential to ovulate) should be evaluated by measuring *FSH*, one of the two hormones that stimulate the ovaries, and *estrogen*, one of the two principal hormones that the ovaries make. Other tests may be used as well to measure ovarian reserve, which is especially important if you are 35 or older. Another area that is essential in your diagnostic workup is an assessment of your pelvic anatomy, especially the fallopian tubes and the uterine cavity. The two most common methods of this evaluation are a *hysterosalpingogram*, an X-ray procedure in which a special iodine-containing solution is injected through the cervix into the uterine cavity to illustrate the inner shape of the uterus and degree of openness of the fallopian tubes, and/or a *laparoscopy*, an outpatient surgical procedure that enables the physician to see all of the pelvic anatomy through a laparoscope inserted into the abdominal cavity.

Seeking Help from an Infertility Specialist

What is most relevant for you and your partner in your beginning medical investigation is to seek the most comprehensive medical care where the physicians are committed to being thorough and efficient. You may already have begun to discuss with your ob-gyn your concerns in conceiving or carrying a pregnancy to term. Some factors may encourage you to remain with your ob-gyn, at least initially, including a positive relationship, proximity to home or work, insurance benefits, and ease in working with office staff.

However, unless your ob-gyn specializes in infertility, works closely with a urologist specializing in infertility, and has established that your diagnosis is straightforward and treatment is not complex, you run the risk of spending money on incomplete or inappropriate diagnostic tests and treatment that may deplete your finances before you are even referred to an infertility specialist (who may require that both of you repeat the very same tests!). Remember that, dedicated as your ob-gyn may be, most of the patients being treated are either pregnant or trying to not become pregnant. Ob-gyns vary in their commitment, training, and ability to provide infertility services. You want (and deserve) to receive specialized care for you and your partner.

Infertility clinics have teams of specialists, such as reproductive endocrinologists, who address both medical and emotional aspects of female and male infertility. These clinics aim to conduct an efficient series of diagnostic tests and a broad range of treatment options 365 days a year. The following factors could mean that the time is right to seek infertility diagnosis and treatment from a specialist:

- If you are under 35 and have been trying to conceive for 12 months; over 35 and have been trying to conceive for more than six months; or over 39 and have been trying to conceive for three months.

- If you or your partner has chronic health problems or a serious past illness. Diabetes, high blood pressure, or a history of cancer are examples of conditions that can affect sperm production and ovarian function.

- If you want to have your diagnostic workup and treatment performed as efficiently as possible with staff, who view "the couple" as the patient, available 365 days a year.

- If you have experienced multiple pregnancy losses.

- If you have been seeing a physician for six months and an infertility evaluation has not been completed.

- If a significant male factor, tubal factor, or moderate or severe endometriosis is identified and in vitro fertilization (IVF) is not available in the practice.

- If procedures such as intrauterine insemination have been attempted or drug therapy such as clomiphene has been prescribed for six cycles or more and no additional testing or treatment has been considered.

- If a fibroid or tubal damage has been noted on a hysterosalpingogram.

- If you report pelvic pain, heavy periods, and/or bowel or bladder symptoms around the time of menstruation, and the physician does not suggest having a hysterosalpingogram or laparoscopy to determine the cause.

The factors above, as well as a belief that you are "stuck" in your infertility rut without further options to pursue, should suggest to you that moving to a higher level of medical care would be appropriate. But disengaging from your ob-gyn can be awkward or difficult, and it is good to be prepared for feelings of ambivalence on both your parts:

"How am I going to tell my gynecologist that I want to go somewhere else for an infertility workup? She tells me that she will be able to do all the tests here in town, and that is certainly tempting, since the nearest (and maybe not even the best) infertility clinic is hours away. I've been seeing her for years, and if I'm lucky enough to get pregnant, I'd like her to deliver our baby. I sure don't want to alienate her over this, but already it has taken months to schedule the initial tests. And the worst part of it is sitting in her waiting room surrounded by pregnant women with their bellies out to here!"

"I'm going crazy with my local ob-gyn. Several of my tests need to be timed to my ovulation cycle, and wouldn't you just know that the day I needed to have blood drawn last month fell on a Sunday, and his office was closed! So now I need to wait another month."

Rather than agonizing about your wish to change to an infertility specialist, a useful strategy would be for you and your partner to meet with your ob-gyn. In this meeting you will want to say something like this: "Dr. Smith, I have asked to meet with you both to thank you for your efforts to treat my infertility and to tell you that Jim and I have decided to seek treatment at the Jackson Infertility Clinic. You have been wonderful in your care and concern for me, but we both know I am getting older, I still am not pregnant, and I want very much to look back on this painful period in my life knowing that I have done everything in my power to seek comprehensive treatment. You have been an important person for me in this process, and I hope I have your support as I move forward. If I do become pregnant, I can't think of anyone I would want to deliver our baby more than you!"

Bringing closure in this way should enable you and your ob-gyn to acknowledge the positive aspects of your work together, even as you are clear that you now want to pursue treatment in a different setting.

Choosing an Infertility Clinic

So you are ready to contact a clinic, but which to choose? There are a few important things to keep in mind, the first two being location and cost. Many clinics provide statistics of "success," but these stats can be easily manipulated. Some clinics take on only low-risk cases, while others count pregnancies that do not develop into healthy fetuses. The statistics that are the most meaningful are those of healthy, live births. It is also helpful to learn the costs associated with infertility procedures, whether the clinic provides counseling or support groups, how they will schedule the timing of tests and procedures for couples coming from a long distance, and whether they will permit your local physician to do some blood tests or injections. You may be able to relate to the following situations:

"I've gone on the Web to check out the nearest infertility clinic. Their statistics are impressive, but somehow it all looks too good to be true. I wish that I could talk to some of their patients to see how satisfied they have been with the treatments."

"The idea of both of us disrupting our lives to travel out of town for treatment is scary. So I made a phone call to one of the clinics and discussed with a counselor just how we could handle all this travel. She said that sometimes blood work and injections can be handled by local doctors and labs who fax the results to the clinic, and that the clinic tries to fit as many tests in for both of us as it can on the day we travel."

Keep in mind that infertility clinics want your business, so it is up to you to tell them what you need in order to decide to become their patient. If getting to the clinic is difficult because of distance, time, cost, or job disruption, propose ways they could make this more manageable. See how flexible they are prepared to be, ask for their suggestions based on other patients like you, and see whether you can make an arrangement that works. The clinic social worker or psychologist may be the best person with whom to have this initial conversation, as those professionals often see their role as being patient advocates. Then pat yourself on the back for being your own effective advocate!

Communicating with Your Partner and Confiding in Others

Many couples keep a tight boundary around their privacy at first, but ultimately it becomes a heavy emotional burden to carry alone. Navigating each person's needs can be difficult, and even talking to one another can be awkward or painful. Here are some examples of situations where couples have found it hard to communicate with each other or with those around them:

"When I told Luke that I wanted to talk with other people about our infertility, he about hit the roof! He thinks this is our private business and he can't understand why I would need to talk to anyone but him about it. So what am I supposed to do at the office when I'm asked to organize a baby shower? Or when I need to come into work late because of blood tests? Or when my best friend, who's pregnant, can't figure out why I'm not all excited about shopping with her for maternity clothes?"

"It came as a real shock to us that Jim is the one who is infertile. My test results seem fine. I almost feel guilty to be the healthy one. But the worst part is that he doesn't want to talk about where we go from here. When the doctor mentioned that I might be able to conceive using artificial insemination with donor sperm, I thought Jim was going to dissolve into the woodwork. I feel like I'm going to burst if I don't talk to someone!"

"My husband just doesn't understand why this is such a big deal for me! If it were up to him, he'd be okay if we never had kids — his hobbies, his job, and his guy friends keep him perfectly happy. I guess he says he wants to begin a family because he knows that will make me happy. But now that I'm miserable, he really doesn't want to hear about it. He keeps trying to jolly me out of my misery. I just want someone who will listen! I really get no comfort from him at all."

Not only do most couples need confidantes beyond themselves, they also need to anticipate how others may react to their news. And they also need to be prepared for the varied and often surprising reactions of others to their news:

"My mom burst into tears when I told her that I was infertile. I think she wants a grandchild every bit as much as I want to have a baby! I can already tell she feels terrible, and I'd give anything not to have to share this kind of news. Frankly, I'm not sure how much I'll be able to lean on her, because my infertility seems to cause her so much pain."

"When I told my sister, I couldn't believe her reaction. Do you know what she said? She has three kids under the age of six, and she told me that if she had it to do all over again, she'd never be a parent! She said I should treasure my vacations, my dinners out, my chance to advance my career, and not make a big deal of not being able to get pregnant! I can't believe she is so unable to understand my pain!"

"Many of our lesbian friends have decided not to become parents. Of course we respect their decision, but we have reached a very different decision for ourselves. We tread rather carefully in deciding how much information to share with these friends about our efforts to become pregnant. Not surprisingly, some are more interested than others about being an informal support network for us."

"My best friend was just wonderful. She let me cry, she brought me books from the library, and she'd always understand that it was a very bad time when I got my period. But as time went on I began to feel a real imbalance in our relationship. She was always eager to be there for me emotionally, but it always seemed as if I was the one leaning on her. Whenever I tried to do something nice for her, she would be awkward about accepting, saying that she knew life was tough for me. After a while I felt that our friendship really was out of balance, and that infertility was to blame."

"My husband tried telling some of his friends about our medical workups, and he was surprised and reassured to learn that almost all of his friends had either known someone who was infertile, who had lost a pregnancy, or who had adopted. He had felt very alone before that, and now he really appreciates his friends asking him about how our infertility workup is progressing."

"My friends have mixed reactions when they hear that I am trying to become pregnant with donor sperm. As a single woman with no plans to marry, I guess I stand out as somewhat unusual among my friends and coworkers, most of whom are either married or divorced. But that's exactly why I need to find out who is sympathetic to my situation, because sometimes I feel as if I'm going to burst with needing to talk! The issues of finding physicians who will take me as a patient; the books of donors and their characteristics; the worry about whether I can be a good parent without a husband — I need to talk about all of these things with friends. I've been lucky to find a good number of people who have been both kind and helpful. But I've also bumped into my share of people with whom I'll never raise the subject of single parenthood again!"

Would a Support Group or Therapist Help?

Many women find that they benefit from being in the company of people who are especially knowledgeable about infertility and its emotional dimensions. For you, this may occur in the early months of diagnosis, or it might occur later during treatment. The two most useful resources that women turn to are support groups and therapists.

Community support groups are available locally, and many are sponsored by the Infertility Awareness Association of Canada (IAAC) or RESOLVE, the national organization in the

US providing public education and information about infertility services. You can also find specialized support groups in clinics across North America where the clinic hires social workers and psychologists to assist patients in discussions about how they are handling the challenges of their infertility. (See the Resources section of this book for organizations that may offer support groups, telephone counseling, or online chat rooms.) A community support group may be right for you if you are comfortable speaking about your personal situation, interested in getting to know other infertile women and men (groups are usually offered to couples, although most groups have more women than men), and if you have questions about local physicians and clinics that other group participants may have used.

Some community support groups allow pregnant women to participate, so if being in a group where some members are pregnant would be distressing for you, ask about this ahead of time. Groups usually meet monthly, and the facilitator may be either a professional or a layperson with a personal history of infertility. Here are some examples of women's experiences with support groups as they were told to me:

"The first time I went to a support group meeting, I really didn't know what to expect. I was determined to keep a low profile. Imagine my surprise when I found that everyone was very welcoming, and that no one expected me to share any personal information other than my first name. I went alone to that first meeting. But since at that point Tom didn't know any guys who were grappling with infertility, and there was a handful of men who attended, I brought Tom to the next one. We both found that the support group was a really strong source of emotional support for us. We became friendly with several of the people in the group and socialized with them. Finally I had a few friends who genuinely understood my misery when I got my period!"

"The support group in my community was good in some ways and not too good in others. The plusses were the lending library and a couple of really solid friendships that I made. But, because I'm not very comfortable speaking up in a group, I didn't participate much in the discussions. It was *very* helpful to hear the experiences of others that paralleled mine, but each month I would leave the group feeling that my shyness held me back from participating as fully as I'd like to."

"The support group I attended was a lifesaver! The members of the group were very forthcoming in talking about their experiences with local physicians, with various infertility clinics, and with how to get a discount on expensive medications. Thanks to the group, I chose a physician who was respectful of her patients and who was willing to spend time with me as we weighed my options. I really benefited from the experiences of women who had gone before me, and I was able to avoid physicians and clinics where the quality of care was lacking."

"You know, I think of myself as someone who could benefit from a support group. I've been in various women's groups and have always gotten a lot out of them. But, unfortunately, the support group in our area had one woman who really monopolized each session. I felt sorry for her, and certainly the members tried to be supportive, but after a few sessions it was clear that she was going to dominate the group, so I stopped attending. At that point in my infertility experience, I needed to be able to give and get support, and the group didn't allow enough of that."

Psychologists and social workers are also available in most communities, either in family service agencies or in private practice. Therapists are ideal if your partner or you do not get as much support as you need from a group, or if you are reluctant to confide personal matters in a group. Therapists are also an excellent choice for women or couples who feel overwhelmed by their infertility, who feel "stuck" in their emotional reactions to their infertility, who are having difficulty talking with others about their needs, and who are having trouble making decisions about treatment, adoption, surrogacy, child-free living, and moving forward with their lives.

Ideally it is best to have a therapist who is familiar with infertility, so that as little time as possible is spent educating the therapist about tests, diagnostic procedures, side effects of medications, and clinic procedures. However, if an informed therapist is not available, then it is especially important to select a therapist who is comfortable and knowledgeable about issues of loss and about couple communication. Those two topics tend to predominate in much of the therapeutic work that infertile women and couples need to do, and a skilled therapist who can address those issues will be a source of support regardless of their level of familiarity with infertility.

You may see a therapist only for a few sessions, while others remain in therapy for months or years, depending on their needs and on how long they have struggled with infertility. The therapy process is different for every woman:

"From the minute I learned that I had a blocked tube, I had such a huge emotional reaction that I knew I needed to see someone who could help me focus on its meaning for my future. My therapist was wonderful, both as an outlet for my stress and as someone who helped me figure out my emotional investment in becoming a parent. We spent some time discussing my feelings of reproductive betrayal before I was ready to make a plan that included some medically invasive procedures. She helped me learn how to be assertive with my doctor, how to guard against letting infertility consume every waking hour, and how to take care of myself emotionally. She really helped me to work 'with' my infertility, rather than to use up lots of emotional energy battling it."

"I was pretty reluctant to see a therapist. Somehow, I'd always thought I should be able to manage my own problems. And I wasn't sure what I should talk about! But my therapist asked some questions that got me started, and as we talked more, I got clearer on the issues that were causing me the most trouble. Some of what we discussed I took home and talked about with Jeff; other issues were more for me to work on. I guess that's one thing I learned about therapy — it's a chance to work on issues that are causing me pain, so those things don't eat away at me. I saw my therapist weekly for a couple of months, and then once a month for the next year or so. By the time we ended I felt as if she had been a real source of support through an emotionally painful time."

"By the time I landed in my therapist's office it was a toss up between a therapist and a divorce lawyer. I know that sounds weird, but life at home had gotten so bad that I wanted out of my marriage. Sam was unwilling to talk about our infertility as much as I needed to talk. He was spending more and more time away from the house, and sex was strictly for baby making. The therapist suggested that Sam and I both come in for some sessions, and that made a tremendous difference in our marriage. We were able to realize how infertility had become a wedge between us — that infertility was the enemy, not each other. Once the therapist helped us to communicate more constructively, Sam and I were finally able to move ahead on decisions about medical options. I can't tell you how glad I am to have gone to a therapist — she really helped to save our marriage!"

"Losing my pregnancy after six months was devastating. A friend suggested a therapist in the community who was comfortable with issues of death and loss. From the moment I met her, I felt as though I could really open up. Although she didn't know much about infertility, she showed such empathy in being able to identify with the pain I was experiencing. She also encouraged me to bring Stu to some of our sessions. He had acted so strong and supportive that I hadn't realized how much he was hurting. Our therapist helped us to grieve together. We made a scrapbook of memories, and this spring we're going to plant a flower garden in memory of Miranda — lots of pink and yellow flowers — the colors we would have used in her nursery. Stu and I are feeling more ready to try for another pregnancy. If I do get pregnant, I'll probably go back to this therapist again, because she really understands why I'll be feeling anxious and apprehensive."

"As a lesbian, I tend to feel different from the mainstream, and I was really concerned about finding a therapist who wouldn't judge me. The person I began seeing is well respected in the lesbian community, even though she only has a basic understanding of the complexities I am facing in trying to get pregnant. But, to her credit, she read some books and articles in an effort to become better informed about the emotional impact of infertility. She and I focused on the 'double whammy' I faced. As a lesbian, I already face a certain awkwardness that arises in the usual office and neighborhood discussions of pregnancy and parenthood, and now that I'm trying to conceive through donor insemination, it's not as if I can cheerfully announce to everyone that I'm trying to get pregnant! So in therapy I'm spending time dealing with the frustration of not getting pregnant, the fear that I might not ever get pregnant, and decisions about how long to keep trying."

Therapists who work with infertile women and their partners can offer some perspectives, such as the following, on who might benefit from therapy:

"I believe that, even though the woman may present herself as the client, it is important for me to meet her partner in an early session, so that I really can think of them as a couple. It is often the case that periodic participation by the partner is advisable, and having met that person early on makes it possible for me to forge a therapeutic relationship with both of them from the beginning."

"In my experience, most infertile clients are in considerable pain when they first arrive in my office. 'I think I'm going crazy!' is often the first phrase that comes out as I ask them how I can help. Once I reassure them that it is natural and expectable to feel so wretched after months or even years of infertility, we often spend the first sessions sorting out where the pain is coming from, how they're dealing with it, and what they want to change. My Kleenex box empties fairly quickly in those early sessions, and I think most clients appreciate that I am here to help them express and then get a constructive grip on their emotions. The clients that can make the best use of therapy tend to be those who can talk about their pain, who are willing to look at their emotions, and who are open to new ways of thinking about and dealing with their current situation."

"As a social worker in an infertility clinic, I tend to see individuals and couples just before or after medical tests and procedures. They are at their most vulnerable when I see them, and we usually focus on how to keep them resilient during the period of diagnosis or treatment. From time to time I find myself serving as an advocate for couples who have not been treated with respect — it's not unusual in a clinic setting for the staff to get caught up in the clinical details of test results and to forget that those test results are being awaited with huge apprehension by the clients. I'm pleased to say that my input has resulted in more sensitivity on the part of clinic staff, but even that sensitivity isn't going to be enough for some couples who get negative test results. So, just as I appreciate feedback from couples who would like us to change some aspects of the clinic, I also appreciate having couples be as clear as possible about how they're handling the stress of infertility. If we start with that as a shared understanding, then usually we can make some progress on finding creative ways of coping."

"I find that clients with infertility will demonstrate a range of reactions: denial, anger, and depression are the most pronounced. I try to acknowledge these reactions and to think through with the client the ways in which they are getting in the way of daily functioning. My preference is for clients to use me as a sounding board for their most compelling feelings, so that they can continue to function in the fertile world outside my office. Once we address emotions, we also can begin to address the decisions that can help the client to move forward. Some of these decisions will involve letting go of hopes and dreams, so I have come to view grief as an integral dynamic with infertile clients."

"I find that most clients come to me hoping that I will be able to 'fix' their pain. What they learn is that we can work together on their pain, but that infertility is a piece of who they are becoming, regardless of the outcome of their diagnoses and treatments. I believe that the couple with infertility needs to learn to stand tall against the world, so I prefer to work with both partners. In doing this I help them with their own communication around painful issues and decisions, while also helping them to appreciate the challenges they must face in communicating with relatives, employers, friends, and neighbors."

Learning to Deal with Infertility

You used to think the word *infertility* applied only to other people, but eventually you start using it more and more frequently. As you use the term with physicians, parents and in-laws, siblings, friends, and coworkers, their reactions will vary. You'll find yourself working as hard at maintaining good relationships as you do at grappling with the medical pathways of infertility. You'll need to correct misinformed people ("No, it isn't our sex life that's to blame." "Medical research says that relaxing has very little to do with conceiving."); be assertive with rude people ("I'm feeling really out of control lately, and I need for you to be more patient with me." "When you make jokes about our infertility, I feel as if you are belittling the hard work that it involves for me."); and educate even supportive friends ("You mean you've never heard of ZIFT?"). As the months pass, you'll know where you can go for support, which people are emotionally available, which medical personnel to turn to for information, and what meaning infertility is assuming in your life. *Infertility* used to be a word you believed would never apply to you, but now the challenge is how infertility will affect you in your quest for parenthood.

Therapeutic Tips

You now appreciate that the initial emotional twinges of frustration and apprehension may be building into more of an upheaval. Some of the issues include deciding when and where to seek more specialized diagnosis and treatment, how to communicate in new ways with your partner, and whom to talk to and how much to tell them. Most importantly, you need to tune in to your emotional self and gauge how much support you need and where to find it. Keep the following points in mind to stay in touch with what's going on with you and your emotions.

- You begin by deciding on an infertility clinic. Although you can do research on the Internet and request material from IAAC and RESOLVE (see the Resources section), it will also be helpful to talk with people in your area who are infertility patients at various clinics. This is easier than you may think. Ask the clinics to contact patients who live in your area and find out if they are willing to talk with you about their experiences. If the clinic intake person hesitates, ask for the name of the clinic psychologist or social worker and see whether that person can help connect you with some local patients. By talking with people who have direct experience with the clinic, you can get vital information that isn't on the stats sheets: whether the clinic is open 365 days a year; whether it offers flexible scheduling, especially for patients coming from a distance; whether it provides patient support groups; whether clinic staff treat patients with respect and compassion; whether doctors review (at regular intervals) the additional medical procedures available if a treatment isn't successful; whether the clinic accepts locally done blood tests; and how satisfied overall the patients are with the care and treatment they receive at the clinic.

- You will notice that your decision of what to tell to whom will evolve over time. In the beginning, as you and your partner are seeking a diagnosis, you may choose to keep your medical details within your immediate family. Later, as you periodically miss work to attend medical appointments, you will decide how open you want to be with supervisors and coworkers who may need to cover for you. And throughout this early process, you will want to talk with your partner about whether and how to seek other sources of emotional support. It is difficult for a couple to bear the emotional burden of infertility alone. The privacy you may need initially can restrict both of you from getting support and new information about local resources. So do consider widening your circle of confidantes and agree on what information you are both comfortable sharing.

- You will want to be careful to keep your relationships in balance. By this, I mean that some friends or relatives, in their empathy for your situation, may begin to relate to you exclusively in terms of your infertility. You will sense that this is happening when conversations with friends open with them asking whether you got your period this month, or how your treatments are going. A simple but effective way of gently steering the relationship back into balance is to thank them for their concern, answer their questions, and then turn the conversation to a mutual topic of interest that has nothing to do with your infertility. Also, remember to take part in the ups and downs your friends are experiencing in their own lives and offer them empathy and support when they need it. This approach will have several additional benefits. First, it will keep you from perceiving yourself as having a scarlet "I" emblazoned on your sweater! Second, it will distract you, even on the most dismal days, from thinking of yourself as being consumed by your infertility — it does not define who you are as a person. And last, it reminds you and others that there are many dimensions to your life.

- You may find, as many women do, that the workplace is one of the most difficult places to coexist with infertility. It is while at work that you may receive a call from the clinic about a failed test result or that your period may begin. At work, people share ultrasound photos, throw baby showers, and bring in their newborns to be admired. If you have told others about your infertility treatments, hopefully they will understand when you have a bad day or when you make yourself scarce during the "oohs" and "ahs" over photographs and infants. But if you are not comfortable sharing your personal information in the work setting, do try to find a coworker who can run emotional interference for you. This person can empathize with you on a bad day, make sure that no one perceives your absence from celebratory events as negative, and steer the topic of conversation away from babies as you join an informal group of your coworkers.

- You should know how to access emotional support from a group or therapist even if you do not initially think that you will need these resources. You may want to attend a local support group meeting at least once to find out whether it feels comfortable and welcoming. One visit will also give you a snapshot of the kind of information and resources the group can connect you with. It is much better to have done your homework and found a good therapist early in the infertility process, so you will have someone available if you need regular emotional support. You, perhaps with your partner, may want to try an introductory visit with a psychologist or a clinical social worker, explaining that you are doing okay for now, but that you would like to check in every so often, and that if and when the stress of infertility mounts you might consider weekly appointments.

Two

The Club:
On the Outside Looking In

As soon as you begin to apply the word *infertility* to your life, the whole world seems filled with pregnant women, mothers and their infants, and babies in strollers. Everywhere you look there are magazine articles on maternity fashions and nursery decorations, books on caring for newborns, TV commercials for baby products and merchandise for the busy mom. Where did all of this come from?

It is also likely that you are feeling especially vulnerable to women who belong to what I call "The Club." These women, pregnant or parenting, rejoice in all things having to do with reproduction and raising children. Club members enthusiastically organize baby showers, delight in comparing notes on their Lamaze classes, offer advice on maternity fashions, consult with one another about difficulties in nursing, and pass around photos of their newborns. They have never given much thought to women with infertility, for whom each baby shower is a poignant reminder of delayed or shattered hopes and dreams.

And although their intent is not to cause you emotional distress, that's exactly what you experience.

It is painful if you have not shared the news of your infertility with Club members, since they will expect you to enthusiastically congratulate friends and coworkers on their pregnancies, participate happily in baby showers, and admire infant photographs. But if you *have* told Club members about your unsuccessful efforts to conceive and your ongoing treatments, you may feel betrayed when they do not recognize the feelings of vulnerability and anger that their activities and conversations provoke in you. This chapter explores the mixed feelings you may have when faced with The Club and gives you helpful coping strategies.

Friends and Coworkers in The Club

Members of The Club are everywhere you go: your neighborhood, workplace, place of worship, and family gatherings. Some will be more invested in their Club membership, and some will be more sensitive to your feelings. However, the challenge you face is in how or whether to coexist with friends and coworkers whose preoccupation with parenthood is consistently a source of anguish for you. You may identify with the following situations that can be very painful to women struggling with infertility:

"Jeff and I learned recently that we'll need to undergo a series of treatments, and even with that the likelihood of my conceiving is only about 30 percent. We've told our parents and our siblings, but I still don't feel comfortable sharing this at work. I'm sure the hormones I'm taking make me even more edgy, but it was all I could do to control my tears as one of my coworkers went flying around the office yesterday announcing her pregnancy. And, wouldn't you know, she got pregnant as soon as she went off birth control! Of course everyone in the office is all excited for her, but I just don't know how I'm going to tolerate the next nine months of her pregnancy and all the fuss it will generate."

"I chose not to attend the baby shower that was held yesterday in the school where I work. The teachers know about my infertility, and they at least had the courtesy to feel awkward about inviting me to the shower. One of my friends promised to defend me if anyone made negative remarks about my absence. I just hate this. Why does everyone have to make such a big deal about a pregnancy? For most of my pregnant friends, it was easy to get pregnant and it was easy to stay pregnant — no big deal. What do they know about those of us who struggle against huge odds just to get pregnant? Can't they understand why this baby shower is like a knife twisting in my heart? Everyone is so ready to share in her joy, but very few people seem to want to understand my pain."

"I'm single and I'm infertile. Most people think it shouldn't be a big deal for me, but what they don't understand is that I want to have a child whether or not I have a partner. So I've begun infertility treatment, but I'm not telling anyone except my closest friends and family. In the meantime, this seems to be the time that everyone in my workplace is either pregnant or a new parent. I can't stand going into the lounge for coffee or for lunch, because all my coworkers talk about is babies. I used to enjoy joking around with these folks, and now all I want to do is keep out of their way."

"I feel so guilty about avoiding my neighbor Fran who is pregnant. I haven't found a way to tell her that it's the pain of my infertility that keeps me from sharing her happiness. She just glows, and I can't bear it. I feel like such a horrible person to be so envious. Is this what infertility does to women — makes us jealous of perfectly nice people whose only crime is that they happen to be pregnant?"

"Although most of my coworkers know my partner, Sandra, the few times I've alluded to becoming a parent 'someday,' people exchange nervous looks, and someone promptly changes the subject. So now that I'm actively trying to become pregnant, I don't feel comfortable sharing this information with folks in the office. But I find myself feeling resentful when I'm expected to join in the fuss over newly pregnant colleagues, especially when I doubt that this same level of congratulations will be extended to me if I'm lucky enough to become pregnant."

"More and more I find myself avoiding spending time with women who are likely to become pregnant. That cuts way down on my friendship network, but I'd rather not begin friendships than distance myself as soon as a pregnant friend begins to show. The mere sight of a woman in maternity clothes is enough to send me to the bathroom to have a good cry. And there would be no rational way of explaining to a friend that I can't bear to be with her because her very physical presence is so devastating. So I'm keeping my friendships with women who are single, menopausal, or who have had their tubes tied. Now how crazy is that?"

Family Members in The Club

Family, whether parents, in-laws, or siblings, is often where we turn for understanding. After all, our families have known us the longest, shared years of our lives, seen us at our best and at our worst, and loved us throughout. Imagine, then, the shock of realizing that some family members are card-carrying members of The Club! These stories tell of women who must cope with their infertility surrounded by their extended family, and they may sound familiar to you:

"I couldn't believe what happened the other day! My sister who already has two kids gave birth to baby number three, and my mother insisted that I go to the hospital to see my newborn niece. Mom knows that Susie's pregnancy was painful for me, she knows that I kept my distance at the baby shower, and she's been good about not talking to me much about her plans for this grandchild. So her insistence that I come to the hospital hit me like a ton of bricks! How can she not know what it will do to me to see dozens of newborns, nursing mothers, doting fathers, and proud grandparents in the maternity ward? How can she not know that a maternity ward, of all places, is where I would most like to be as a new mother? How can she not know that being there as an infertile woman is too much to ask of me? My own mother — I feel so betrayed!"

"In our family, christenings are a big event. They're an excuse for us to come together and an opportunity for distant relatives to see the new babies for the first time. (The children get a kick out of counting how the kids are beginning to outnumber the adults.) This week when I told my sister that I wouldn't be attending because I didn't feel genuinely able to participate in the joyfulness, it was as if I had driven a knife into her heart. Here she has the entire family prepared to focus on her and the baby, and now she has decided to make a big deal of my absence. I'm only asking to be spared the misery of one more event that focuses on babies — yet she insists on seeing this as my refusal to rejoice in her baby. I keep trying to tell her it's the event, not the baby, but she just doesn't get it. She has a lot of nerve complaining to me, when she's the one with the baby and I'm the one with empty arms."

"My sister has had a tough life, and I've tried to stick by her through thick and thin. Our parents were killed in a car accident several years ago, and now we're pretty much the only family left except for some really distant relatives. Her marriage has been rocky from the start and after her husband left her six months ago, she discovered that she was pregnant. That felt like such an irony, since my marriage is solid as a rock and I've been unable to get pregnant for the past four years. Anyway, I've been providing a shoulder for her to lean on while she picks up the pieces of her life. She knows about my sadness in not being able to get pregnant, but what happened yesterday shows me how she has no clue about my emptiness. With great excitement, she announced to me that, even though I couldn't have a baby of my own, she wanted for me to help her have her baby — she wants me to coach her through childbirth! I was so staggered that I just told her I'd think it over, and I left. Then it hit me: here I'd be learning Lamaze techniques with her in a room full of pregnant women, going to the hospital, and spending hours on the maternity ward with crying infants and starry-eyed new parents. I know I cannot be her labor coach, but now I'm furious that it's up to me to figure out how to explain this to her. I assumed all along that she understood the pain my infertility causes me. For her to think that she can soothe this pain by having me as her coach is just beyond belief!"

"My brother hasn't spoken to me for the past month — and all because I sent my gift to the baby shower instead of coming to the shower myself. What does he want from me? Here his wife gets pregnant after only a couple months of trying, she sails through her entire pregnancy without so much as a bit of morning sickness, she has a roomful of happy friends and relatives at the shower, and all he can focus on is that I chose not to attend. His attitude is that my infertility shouldn't prevent others from taking pleasure in their pregnancies — fine. But it doesn't mean that I have to be in the front of the cheering section. I'm furious that he doesn't understand, I'm furious that he's making this such a big deal when he should be looking forward to his baby's birth, and I'm furious that infertility has the power to cause so much conflict between people who love each other."

"My husband, of all people, just doesn't get it. The other day he said to me that he wants me to stop focusing so much on the devastation of my infertility and to get back in the swing of life again. He's tired of treading on eggshells, worrying about what will set me off on a crying jag or whose insensitivity has made me furious. He says that, as much as he wants a baby, he has come to realize that he wants it mostly so that I will be happy. For me, his message is that he only wants me to show him positive emotions and just to stifle all the other emotions that are such a big part of infertility. I thought we were going through this together. Now it seems that if I'm going to feel unhappy or upset, he doesn't want any part of it."

Creative Coping

Members of The Club are likely curious about your family situation, and sometimes their inappropriate responses to your childlessness are enough to make you consider life in a convent. How do you cope? Where do you seek solace? Undoubtedly you will turn to your partner (see Chapter 1 for the pitfalls here, Chapter 3 for partner communication strategies, and Chapter 5 for how to restore intimacy to your relationship) and likely to your family (see this chapter and Chapter 6 for the unanticipated insensitivities of family members). But you must also remember to seek out your inner strength and find ways to deal with Club members around you.

Women deal with the pain of their infertility in many ways, and the theme of avoidance runs through the voices of the women on these pages. And although avoidance is certainly an understandable response, there are other ways of dealing with the fertile world that may produce more positive feelings for you:

"I decided from the beginning that I would try to talk about how I needed support in new ways from my friends and coworkers. So, bless them, everyone in the office has been really good about reaching out to me — I have to ask, but when I ask, they're there. They understand that when I say I got my period that morning, it's another month down the drain and another reminder that I'm not pregnant. They understand that it's too painful for me to join in discussions of babies and pregnancies, so someone will tactfully change the subject if I walk in on that kind of conversation. I'm really very lucky to have such good coworkers, and I tell them in lots of ways how their thoughtfulness eases my pain."

"My friends' pregnancies coincided with learning that Greg and I are infertile. I had to decide how I wanted to connect with my pregnant friends who were so joyful at a time that my heart was aching. It really came down to individuals. A few of my pregnant friends just couldn't contain themselves, they were so preoccupied with every detail of their pregnancies. I told those friends that since their pregnancies were such a big part of their lives that I couldn't share, I wouldn't be seeing as much of them as earlier. In fact, they had already begun to gravitate toward those people who would dote on them, so our parting was fairly mutual. With other pregnant friends, I openly discussed how I valued their friendship, but how I would need to ask for special consideration: not discussing their pregnancy with me, not inviting me to their baby showers, not expecting me to visit while the baby was still an infant. That's been delicate, but it has worked out reasonably well. Their thoughtfulness tells me that our friendship matters. I'm eternally grateful at their willingness to let me share parts of their lives, but I can't share the parts that involve their babies."

"Although I didn't set out to befriend infertile women, they're actually the closet network of friends that I have these days. We definitely have issues in common, and there's no need to explain much about diagnostic tests, medical procedures, hormones, treatments, and feelings of hopelessness. The good thing about being friends with other women who are infertile is that there's a real reciprocity. My fertile friends are always afraid to complain to me about their lives because they feel as if their complaints are trivial compared to mine — and they're mostly right! But my infertile friends and I have a rhythm in supporting one another. One week someone gets her period or has bad test results and she leans on me. The next week I've had to put up with an office baby shower, and she's there for me. And even though it will be painful if one of my infertile friends gets pregnant, there's something to be said for knowing what she went through to have her dream come true. At some level, I guess I also believe that if it could happen to her, maybe it could happen to me."

Getting Support from Club Members

Dealing with members of The Club can be frustrating, but if you are inclined, you can seize the opportunity to help them understand how they can support you. In communicating about your infertility, it is best if you speak in terms of what the other person can do to be supportive, rather than how miserable you are feeling. Here are some of the ways that women have communicated their needs to Club members:

"Expecting me to participate in events with pregnant women and little babies is asking too much at a time when I don't know if I will ever be able to get pregnant or to cradle my baby in my arms."

"I don't mind at all if people change conversation topics when I walk into the room. I'd much rather have that happen than be stuck in conversation about life events that I may never be able to enjoy."

"If you're not sure how I will react to something, just ask. For me, I get along fine with toddlers, but infants just bring tears to my eyes. Baby showers are okay these days, but do not ask me to come over to see the baby when it's still little."

"As for learning about someone's pregnancy, I'd prefer to hear it quietly from one person at the end of the day, so I can go home and make myself a soothing cup of tea and nurse my feelings of envy in solitude."

"When I tell you that I just got my period, it means much more than that. It means the treatment has not been successful this month, it means I'm not pregnant, it means I will have to spend more money and endure more disruption continuing the treatment, and it means that I'm one month older without a pregnancy and not getting any younger. It would be nice for you to say that you're sorry and to ask what we can do together that would be soothing."

The Club is a source of such mixed emotions. You resent its existence, but you also wish that you could join and show off photos of your ultrasound or your chosen child, accept baby gifts and hand-me-downs, and revel in the adoration that will be heaped upon your baby after not just months, but years, of waiting to welcome this new family member.

But the reality is that during your period of infertility you will bear the burden of educating other people who are caught up in their own parenting world, specifying for them how they can be supportive and also excluding some of them from your life. There are times this burden seems to be too much, and there are other times you hope that your messages will sensitize them so that others "looking in" will not feel so misunderstood. Most important is the realization that, should you ever have a child, you will be in the best position to offer sensitive behavior and responses to other women who yearn for a baby to cuddle in their arms.

Therapeutic Tips

Club membership is a given for many of our friends and family members, but you still have choices about how and whether you continue your relationships with these folks. As you already have discovered, membership doesn't define the individual — empathy does. So here are some categories of empathy, ranging from supportive to incorrigible,

with my suggestions of how (or whether) to include these
Club members in your life:

- **Supportive:** These individuals are capable of empathizing
  with your infertility and your efforts to cope with it. Take
  them into your confidence, and explain what kind of support and friendship would be most helpful to you these days.
  Also, explain that as time passes you may need to revise your
  requests for support, since you know infertility has already
  changed your life and will continue to have an impact on
  you that you can't foresee. Explain that you are trying not
  to define yourself in terms of your infertility, and that you
  hope your relationship can be filled with fun and mutual
  supportive understanding.

- **Clueless:** These individuals either haven't made the effort
  to think through how infertility is shaping your life, or they
  simply aren't interested in trying. You can check out whether
  they are capable of making a genuine effort to understand the
  challenges of your infertility and to be emotionally supportive. If you decide that someone won't respond with empathy,
  you have several options. Minimizing contact with the person
  is one choice, and asking for a sympathetic loved one to run
  interference for you is another. A final option is communicating with the person, face-to-face or in writing, to alert the
  person to what you hope and expect by way of sensitivity.

- **Incapable:** These individuals either do not give priority to
  your emotional needs or are so self-involved that their own
  needs will always override yours. I suggest writing a letter clarifying your situation. The purpose of this letter is to
  educate, request support, express that infertility need not
  come between you, and clarify that you are making careful
  decisions to gather around you friends and loved ones who

can be supportive. This letter may evoke a range of responses, and you can decide how or whether to pursue your relationship with each person based on how they react.

- **Incorrigible:** These individuals refuse to be supportive of you and expect you to meet *their* needs, which will make you feel guilty or angry. Once you determine that someone falls into this category, protect yourself from their manipulative and selfish behavior. If possible, minimize all but the most essential contact with that person, and have an escape plan if any contact with this person upsets you.

Three

Emotional Overload:
Staying Together through Infertility

Even as you feel overwhelmed by your own infertility experience, your partner is living this experience too, but with a different perspective and different worries, apprehensions, and preoccupations. Although you share the same experiences, you each may take away distinctly different messages. And that is another of the many challenges of infertility: how can you and your partner work through this unwanted life event without succumbing to the stress?

Women who are trying to conceive may be married, in a committed lesbian relationship, single with a close partner, or single without a partner. Although there will be some overlap in the responses that partners demonstrate to infertility, in this chapter I will offer a separate segment for the reactions of husbands and a separate segment for the reactions of non-birthing partners in lesbian relationships. Also, I will offer my clinical perspective on why a partner may be responding to infertility in a particular way, based on what

I have learned from my interactions with hundreds of infertile couples.

Single women, whether straight or lesbian, hopefully will have a social network of friends and relatives to support them in their efforts to conceive, during their pregnancies, and when they later give birth and begin their new roles as single parents. Although this chapter does not address their issues from a partner perspective, it undoubtedly captures many of their emotions as women hoping to become mothers.

Partners can be a comfort, a frustration, a source of strength, a disappointment, a source of empathy, or an emotionally remote housemate. The crisis of infertility tests a relationship in new ways, and couples must find creative strategies to discuss and resolve unanticipated dilemmas. You should know that counselors and support groups can provide new ways of looking at your situations, which can enable you to cope differently and more effectively. Hopefully the voices in this chapter will remind you that you are not alone in the ways you grapple with infertility, and perhaps some of the examples will suggest new ways of comforting, coping, and finding the emotional resilience to face the treatments and decisions that lie ahead.

Husbands

Husbands' responses to the infertility that they are encountering will differ greatly, and their responses will change over time. However, the following statements by husbands and the responses of wives demonstrate that some key issues come up again and again:

The husband says: "I want a baby as much as she does, but I can't let my feelings get the best of me."

The wives say:

"I can't believe that he'll come home from work, see that I'm down in the dumps, and just ignore my misery and start a conversation about something from his day. When I tell him that I've gotten my period or that someone in my office is pregnant, he'll spend maybe a minute on it and then change the subject. So I bring him back to the source of my misery for the day and tell him how I *feel* about it. Now I can understand that he might not be able to share my distress at another office pregnancy, but surely he should also feel distressed at my getting my period instead of getting pregnant. It took a long time before I could even get him to admit his sadness each time I get my period. It's clear that I need to lead the way by exposing my feelings, because he's just not into talking about his."

"My husband has always been really supportive of me no matter what I'm trying to do. So when the infertility workup began it didn't surprise me that he was supportive. But after a while it began to feel one-sided, since I'd always be the upset one and he'd always be the calming influence. The longer this went on the crazier I began to feel. When I asked him if I was the only one who felt bummed out by all the frustrations of our infertility, at first he made light of it. But the longer we talked about our dream of having a baby and how that just wasn't happening, I could see that he was sad, but that his way of handling sadness was to distract himself by comforting me. So we made a deal, because I told him I couldn't stand being the only one of us who expressed emotions. We agreed that whenever he comforted me, he would also talk about how the event or issue was affecting him. That way

I could also take a turn at comforting him. It isn't always easy, but it's much better to try to be equal emotional partners in this infertility struggle."

"For the longest time I believed that our infertility was affecting me emotionally more than it was him. Lots of times we just would ignore the whole emotional thing and focus on the logistics of doctors' appointments, the side effects of my medications, and how our savings was disappearing with every month of treatment. Then one day we were in the park and I left him for a couple of minutes to go to the restroom. When I came out, I could see that his attention was completely absorbed by watching a father teach his little boy how to pitch a baseball. As I got closer I could see that Bill was wiping tears from his eyes. I just put my arms around him and we both had a good cry right there in the park. That was the beginning of his willingness to talk with me about the grief that he feels at not becoming a father. I think it's hard for him to feel these emotions, but it's definitely helped me to feel more connected to him now that he is willing to talk about how he feels."

Many husbands feel responsible for helping *you* through this difficult time. However, a challenge in the long term is that he will stifle his own feelings (as males have been so well socialized to do) and try to support you, but refuse to acknowledge that he, too, feels a sense of impending loss. Your role, then, in addition to being aware of your own emotions, is to encourage your husband to share *his* feelings about infertility. In that way, you are both in a better position to talk together, rather than having him believe that he belongs solely in a supportive role. Frankly, for some husbands, it is far more comfortable to be in that supportive role, because it doesn't expose their vulnerability.

But constant support is a heavy load to carry for any one person, so do what you can to learn the ways in which you and he can be mutually supportive. And don't hesitate to seek out a therapist to help you if you get stuck.

The husband says: "I don't know how to help her through this."

The wives say:

"I'll tell you what really used to make me feel as if he and I lived on different planets. I would be in tears about something related to our infertility and he would try to cheer me up! After this had happened a bunch of times, I finally said to him that I needed for him to just shut up and hold me on his lap. I must have cuddled with him and cried for about ten minutes. Then I wiped my eyes, got up and washed my face, and thanked him for just holding me quietly. He asked if that really helped, and when I told him it was much better than having him try to cheer me up, he looked so confused! So we talked about it, and it was then that the light bulb went off in my head: he wasn't a mind reader. I needed to tell him how he could help me, otherwise he'd just muddle on and probably get it all wrong. Things have been much better since then, and I've gotten past my belief that he was an insensitive oaf who couldn't soothe my pain!"

"I can't tell you how many times my husband has responded to a negative piece of infertility news by proposing that we get out of town for the weekend. When I would say that I couldn't possibly have a good time after the news we'd just gotten, he would assure me that we needed to keep life in perspective and not lose our ability to have fun. So we'd sit down, plan a camping trip or a visit with his brother in the city, or take a hike in the local park. And I'd drag myself along and try to get in the spirit of things. But it never worked. Finally I told him that we needed to find a different way to put life in perspective, because running away from my feelings was making me feel as if I carried a burden along with me on each of our trips. He had sensed that I wasn't getting any pleasure out of our 'escapes,' but it wasn't until I insisted that we handle it differently that we finally talked about how to handle his feelings and mine better. I told him that I need to talk, and maybe to cry and yell, about how rotten I feel each time another month passes, each time another medical result comes back, and each time another friend gets pregnant. We discussed for a while whether I should go into counseling. But before going that route we agreed that we'd reserve 15 minutes a day to talk about our infertility. We could stretch to longer on days when really upsetting things happened, but we agreed that 15 minutes should mostly be enough time. What my husband and I discovered was that in those 15 minutes we *both* ended up talking, we both ended up understanding each other's perspectives, and we both felt better connected to how infertility was affecting our lives. He said that the 'let's get out of town' routine was to protect us from being overwhelmed by our infertility, but now that we talk, vent, problem solve, and grieve more together, we're both more able to feel as if we're taking things in stride. And when we do get out of town, I don't feel as if we're running away, but instead, as if we're taking a break that we both need."

"My husband, who is something of a computer nerd, took great comfort in being able to search the Internet for medical information, to make tables of my treatments and the side effects of my meds, and even spreadsheets of the costs we have had to pay out of pocket for our infertility. So why should I have been surprised that every time I began talking about infertility, he booted up his computer? On some level it was nice to know that *one* of us was coping, but after a while it was clear to me that all these facts and figures weren't beginning to touch my sadness and frustration. So that's what I told him, and the poor guy just looked so puzzled. He thought all of his hard work had been soothing to me. I just plain told him that I needed for us to talk about how the infertility was affecting our marriage and our emotions as a couple. To be honest, we didn't get very far, since he was so worried that I was about to bail out on the marriage, and I was so sad that I couldn't talk very coherently. And then, when I suggested counseling, he really got worried! But we were lucky in finding a great counselor who was suggested by a friend who is infertile. And to our surprise, she was able to strike lots of responsive chords as she asked questions about the impact that infertility was having on our lives. By talking with her we learned better ways of communicating with each other. And I'm relieved to say that the computer isn't used for much infertility stuff any more, so it is no longer a refuge for my husband or a roadblock for me."

Remember, husbands are not mind readers, and they are unlikely to know how to be supportive unless you tell them. It terrifies them to see their wives feeling sad, frustrated, and tense. They may respond by trying to ignore bloodshot eyes, changing the subject, submerging themselves in their hobbies or work, or trying to distract you with irrelevant stories or jokes. Few husbands appreciate that "just" holding and cuddling their wives may be immensely comforting. With their focus on procedures and test results, they may not understand why quoting statistics is not a source of hope and consolation to their wives, who may be preoccupied with other events like the beginning of their period or a negative piece of news from the doctor. Because men often believe that they should be able to "fix this" or "make her feel better," many husbands are doomed to feel that they are failing in the relationship.

It will be important to communicate that your sadness has to do with your infertility and not with his inability to make you happy. Along with that, be sure to convey whatever you can about what he can do to be helpful and supportive as infertility erodes your good cheer, your hopefulness, and your confidence that you will conceive and have a healthy pregnancy. And, while you're at it, remember to ask *him* what you can do to ease his pain and to keep your relationship on course.

The husband says: "Infertility is taking its toll on our marriage."

The wives say:

"You know, there's no question our marriage has felt like it's under siege. Neither of us expected that something like trying to have a baby could be such a source of stress. I think one of the worst things is that both our time and our money are being consumed by infertility. It would be one thing if we could be sure that all of this would result in a baby, but there are no guarantees. So we spend less money on ourselves, work overtime, and take modest vacations once a year. We both feel sad that our lives are on hold, and that we do fewer and fewer fun things together."

"After having been married for six years and carefully practicing birth control, it came as a rude jolt when I didn't get pregnant as soon as we decided to begin our family. Our reason for waiting these six years was so that we could do it right — we both got the educations we needed for our jobs, we both moved up in our professional positions, and we bought a house in a good school district. I guess we thought we were in control of our destinies until we bumped into this infertility mess. And that's what it feels like — a mess! I'm taking hormones, and that leads to mood swings on top of the depression I'm already feeling. My husband is spending more and more time at work, because we know the costs of traveling to and from the infertility clinic will mount up. And frankly, I'm no fun to be around when he is home. I guess we're just not very good at taking in stride the biggest upset of our lives."

"We decided to begin a family right after we got married, since we were both in our mid-thirties and we knew our chances of conceiving wouldn't get better with time. Well, that's an understatement! It's been three years now, and we're both beginning to wonder if our marriage can withstand the sadness of not having a baby. It's been really hard on both of us, being newly married and grappling with the worry of infertility. I envy the couples in our support group who seem to know how to comfort one another, how to disagree without it escalating into World War III. Brian and I have had to learn how to be a married couple with the cloud of infertility hanging over us every minute. It's hard to remember the fun times we had before we were married, and it's impossible to plan for any fun times with ovulation cycles, blood tests, and ultrasounds taking up so much of my life. Brian feels like an injured bystander, since he knows there's nothing he can do to improve my chances of conceiving."

"I can't believe how infertility has wrecked our sex life! We keep a calendar downstairs with my days of ovulation marked on it, and when the ovulation kit says 'Go!' we give it a half-hearted try. Let me tell you, baby making bears no resemblance to lovemaking. These days it's sex on schedule. We've tried having sex at other times of the month, but what's the use? I can't even remember the last time I felt sexually aroused. Who could have imagined that infertility would rob us of our erotic feelings for one another?"

Infertility takes a toll on marriages in myriad ways. Ultimately, it is up to both of you (perhaps with the help of a therapist) to talk about ways that you can grieve together, communicate more clearly, deal with the disruptions of infertility treatment, cope with the financial costs, separate lovemaking from baby making, and shape your future together. It is not so much infertility that hurts marriages as it is the demands it places on the couple for emotional flexibility and resilience.

However, it sometimes happens that one partner is fertile and decides that being a birth parent is more important than staying with an infertile partner. In this case, it's common for the infertile person to offer to let the fertile partner out of the marriage. (Perhaps this is an important discussion for the couple to have up-front, so they can reaffirm what is important in their lives.) The infertile partner may offer this openly, or may even attempt to drive the other person away by sabotaging the marriage through hurtful words or behavior. In the end the fertile partner may indeed decide to leave the marriage — not because of infertility, but because the couple never knew what the struggle to become parents really meant to their relationship. Once again, communication is the key to sorting out the complexities of infertility in your marriage.

The husband says: "I don't even care anymore if we have a baby. I just want her to be happy again."

The wives say:

"I can't believe that after all these years of infertility treatment, he's ready to give up! I know that in the beginning we both desperately wanted to have a baby. And I've been the one who has had to adjust the most to the medical interventions — the toll on my body and moods, the interruptions in my work schedule, the inability to plan ahead. I've tried hard to choose the right doctors, the right clinics, the right procedures. And now he wants to throw all that away? It seems as if he is saying that he wants to have me happy again so that our marriage can get back on track, and I'm saying that I want to have a baby so that our marriage can get back on track."

"Not only has infertility changed me, it has changed our entire view of what it is to be a couple. I had always thought that being a couple came first, and building a family came next. Chad had agreed with that perspective, but somewhere along the line he began to question whether the struggle to build a family was worth the toll it was taking on me and on our relationship. We really felt stuck in a cycle of two weeks of waiting to see if I got my period and then two more weeks of hoping that I'd be able to conceive *this time* I ovulated. Finally we began asking ourselves whether the quest for a baby was robbing us of our pleasure in life. So now we are sitting down to decide whether we could be happy going through life without children. If the answer to that question is 'no,' then I think we may be ready to ask ourselves whether adopting a baby would be a different pathway to our happiness as a family. I don't know where these conversations will land, but it feels better to have them than to be stuck."

"When my husband began to question whether or not we should continue our infertility treatment, which had proved so emotionally exhausting for both of us, we decided to take a three-month 'vacation.' That was a really difficult decision to reach, because we'd lose precious months. But we had to know how it felt to have our lives back without infertility being on our minds every minute. So we notified the clinic that we would consider resuming treatment in three months, we told our therapist that we would call her if we needed her, and we planned some time out of town so we could be away from all the familiar reminders of our infertility struggle — including well-meaning friends and family. We needed to see if we could get our lives back. I guess we also needed to see if we still felt complete as a couple, since so much of our time in the past few years had been spent talking about how we would feel complete once we had a baby."

This final statement by the husband speaks poignantly to the toll that infertility can take, and to the sad recognition that the relationship will never again be the same. This husband clearly feels that the quest for parenthood has exacted too great a cost — he wants to preserve what he can of the marriage and, once again, he is looking for a way to "fix" his wife's sadness. Since men in North American society are not socialized toward parenthood in the same way that women are, it is easier for some of them to look to other rewarding life choices that do not include parenthood. However, a husband's willingness to forgo parenthood will probably offer little consolation to his wife. The two of them need to find ways of reintroducing some pleasure into their lives, and ultimately they need to decide how long and to what ends they will pursue their efforts to become parents.

Lesbian Partners

If you are in a lesbian relationship, you know that many factors have shaped your decision to seek assistance in conceiving a baby. Chances are that you both have given careful consideration to which of you will try to become pregnant first, and you hope you can conceive quickly!

Lesbians enter the path to parenthood with what has been called *social factor infertility*, whereby their choice of a female partner prevents them from conceiving without a sperm donor. Some lesbians will conceive through intercourse, some will self-inseminate with sperm from a known donor, and many will seek the assistance of a physician who is supportive of their desire to conceive. Others will use the services of an infertility clinic, with assurance that advanced technology will be available and that clinic hours on weekends and holidays will allow them to be inseminated at the time of ovulation.

Lesbian couples who have trouble conceiving will experience many of the same issues as heterosexual couples. Impatience, frustration, and sadness accompany the hope and anticipation of any couple using assisted reproductive technology. However, lesbians also face unique challenges when seeking medical help to conceive. First, some health-care professionals will behave awkwardly when accepting a lesbian as an infertility patient. Second, many clinic questionnaires are designed on the assumption the patient is in a heterosexual relationship, so that may feel off-putting. And finally, as you may already have experienced, clinic staff may be confused about your relationship (sisters? best friends?). Only you can decide whether the convenience and quality of medical care make it worthwhile to stay in a clinic that is not gay-friendly. And even though the power relationship between patients and physicians can deter you from being openly critical, you may be able to encourage your physician to sensitize the clinic staff so all patients feel welcome.

These medical barriers mean that lesbians must select physicians and infertility clinics that appreciate the unique circumstances of lesbians hoping to conceive. And as a lesbian couple hopes for a successful pregnancy, their anticipation is tempered by the reality that the partner of the birth mother will not be legally accepted as a mother, but will need to go through the legal formality of adopting the baby.

The following statements demonstrate some of the unique challenges facing lesbian couples, with examples of how each partner might react:

The non-birthing partner says: "Once we decided we wanted to have a baby, our next decision was 'which of us will try to become pregnant?'"

The birthing partners say:

"This was an interesting challenge, since both of us are in good health and both of us felt really positive at the prospect of being pregnant. Ultimately we resolved the question by reminding ourselves that our long-term plans were to have more than one child, so hopefully each of us would have the opportunity to be a birth mother. We decided for baby number one that I would try to become pregnant, in part because I have better health insurance and I have more flexibility to work from home."

"We asked at our clinic whether I could pursue IVF, using donor sperm and my partner's eggs. In that way I would be the gestational surrogate of my partner's baby, and both of us would feel that we were sharing conception in a very special way. The clinic agreed, so that's our solution to pursuing motherhood!"

"Since my partner has several health problems that would be aggravated by becoming pregnant, we both hoped that I would be successful in conceiving. We decided that she would be the stay-at-home mom after I delivered, so in that way both of us would have important experiences in parenting our baby."

"I always have wanted to be pregnant and to nurse a baby. Jan is open to the idea of being a birth mother, but she was really very willing for me to try first to conceive. We agreed that if I didn't get pregnant after a year, she would be glad to try to conceive. Our real priority has always been on becoming parents, and who carries the pregnancy is not especially important."

Once the couple reaches the decision to pursue parenthood, lesbians face both the questions of "who?" or "who first?" and also the fortunate opportunity for the other partner to try to conceive if the first partner's attempts are not successful. They both will share in the suspense of whether or when a pregnancy will occur, but there are a variety of creative answers to the question of who will be the birth mother.

The non-birthing partner says: "How are we going to arrange for you to get pregnant?"

The birthing partners say:

"I would like for us to choose someone we know to be the sperm donor. We've both talked with several of our guy friends, and once we narrow it down we'll decide on the details. I'm not interested in having intercourse, so once one of our friends agrees to donate his sperm, I'll just use a turkey baster, which worked fine for several lesbian couples we know. I know it sounds weird, but it allows me to bypass the whole clinic insemination routine."

"My partner hopes that her brother would be willing to donate his sperm, so when I conceive at least some of her family DNA will be in our baby. That's fine with me, since I know her brother and think of him as a really fine person. I'd like to inseminate myself, but if that doesn't work, I'd consider having intercourse once we pinpoint my most fertile time of the month."

"I have decided to ask my gynecologist to perform intrauterine insemination (IUI) using donor sperm from a sperm bank. Since my partner and I hope eventually to have more than one child, we plan to arrange for some of this donor's sperm to remain frozen so we can use it again when we try to conceive our first baby's siblings."

For lesbian couples planning to use sperm from a known donor, it will be important to be clear about whether, or to what extent, the donor will relate to the baby after its birth. Just as the non-birthing mother will need legally to adopt the baby of her partner, both mothers should seek legal clarification and documentation about the role the sperm donor will have in their lives and the life of the baby. Some families are eager to have the donor very involved; others prefer that the donor remain a family friend, and still others want to be sure that he understands his role with their family has been strictly as a donor — nothing more. And for those women using frozen sperm from a sperm bank there is the opportunity to select a donor with characteristics that have a special appeal to the prospective mothers.

The non-birthing partner says: "It has been a whole new experience facing the non-gay-friendly environment of the infertility clinic."

The birthing partners say:

"After filling out all the forms asking for 'husband's name,' 'husband's urologist,' and various other questions, I just took a red pen and crossed through those questions. When a staff member asked me why I hadn't answered, I explained that I have a female partner and the questions do not relate to us. She said 'oh,' and disappeared. So when I saw the doctor, I mentioned how the intake form seemed inappropriate for same sex couples and, to my surprise, he asked if I would be willing to revise the form so it was more user friendly to all patients, including single women. Since I'm sure I'm going to be spending lots of hours in their waiting rooms, I said I'd give it a try. But, honestly, I feel pretty good about his recognition of the problem I posed and his willingness to consider a solution."

"When I was called into the exam room, the attendant asked me if my husband would be available to talk to the doctor after the exam. I asked if she had read my records, and when she said she had not, I told her that I have a lesbian partner who is in the waiting room and who would like to be in the examining room with me. She looked a bit flustered, said she would check, and disappeared. When the doctor arrived, I explained that I had asked the nurse if my partner could be present during my exam, but I hadn't received an answer. The doctor consulted the chart, asked if my partner's name was Cheryl Sutton, and when the nurse arrived a moment later, asked her to show my partner into the room. I then said to the doctor how nice it would be if clinic staff could be alerted that not all patients are heterosexual, and asked what the clinic does to help its staff be sensitive to diversity in its patients. He paused, said he hadn't given it much thought, but he agreed that it would be worth raising at a staff meeting. Cheryl was shown into the room at that point, only to hear me offering to make a presentation at any staff meeting where the topic was on the agenda! If I don't get an invitation in a month or two, I think I'll repeat my offer and see if I can make any headway."

"Once again I find myself frustrated and angry to be in a clinic where I'm assumed to be heterosexual. Not only did an intake worker ask me if my husband's urologist had forwarded his records, but the look of awkward confusion at my answer convinced me that I'm probably the first lesbian she has knowingly met."

These and other examples demonstrate that some infertility clinics have staff who are unfamiliar with how to make same sex couples feel comfortable and accepted in an environment that for so many years offered its services to married couples. For those patients who choose to be assertive, there is always the possibility that their offers to help will be solicited or accepted. For those patients who encounter inappropriate or rude behavior, a written complaint to the personnel office would be a logical response. If the clinic has a psychologist or a social worker on staff, it would be reasonable to meet with them to discuss your concerns about the lack of respect you feel in the clinic, and what has contributed to that feeling. Those helping professionals, who often see themselves as patient advocates, may be in the best position to address your concerns from the inside of the organization. However, if you find yourself clenching your teeth in silence, rather than drawing attention to slights or rude treatment, you probably are in the throes of a power imbalance. Not only are you depending on the staff to help you get pregnant, but you also would like that to happen as cooperatively as possible. For you, an anonymous letter to the personnel department or a counselor on staff may be the closest you want to come to making a complaint. And that is understandable, given that you really want the focus to be on a successful pregnancy. It is always a challenge to weigh the roles we assume in various settings, and you have a right to decide where you want your focus to be as you concentrate on your efforts to conceive. Just keep in mind that, over time, different options may seem more plausible as you become more familiar with the clinic, its staff, and the best ways of requesting flexibility in behavior.

The non-birthing partner says: "Whenever I get my period, which is no big deal, I worry that maybe this month Chris will get her period too, and that will be a sad time and another lost month for us."

The birthing partners say:

"Getting my period was bad enough before I began intrauterine insemination. The week or so of PMS, the cramps, and the general discomfort were no picnic. But now my period has such a symbolic meaning of loss. Kelly can sense my PMS almost before I do, and we both begin to have a premonition that this is not the month to celebrate a pregnancy. It is really a comfort to have someone who is so in tune with my biological rhythms. I only hope that she can share those rhythms in a different way when I get pregnant."

"It's so strange to be so aware of my period. Since Jan is the one who has cramps and mood swings, we would both be on high alert when she got her period because she felt so rotten. Now we both feel rotten when we get our periods, since mine represents the non-pregnancy. We've decided to indulge ourselves when we get our periods, just as a way of not letting them get us down too much. So the first day of a period is now an excuse to go out for dinner or a nice dessert, or maybe to pick up a colorful bouquet at the florist. We both know we're trying to get past the sadness for me and the discomfort for her, but so far it's working pretty well."

Unlike the experience of heterosexual couples, there's no question about a lesbian partner being unable to understand the meaning of her partner getting her period! The significance of another month passing without a pregnancy is heightened for females who are so in tune with one another's biological rhythms.

The non-birthing partner says: "It has been strange to face the reaction of our families to the news that Sharon is trying to get pregnant."

The birthing partners say:

"Our families' reactions were directly parallel to their acceptance of us as lesbians. Marilyn's parents have welcomed me from the start and have been clear that they cherish me because I make their daughter happy. So it was no surprise to hear their happiness when we announced our plans to conceive their grandchild. No fuss from them about the fact that the baby would have none of their genes — just hopes for a healthy pregnancy and a healthy birth. They've even offered to help with the costs of the inseminations. My parents, on the other hand, have always believed that I would 'come to my senses' someday, and they've avoided references to my lifestyle as much as possible. They're clearly uncomfortable around Marilyn, and she and I keep any visits with my parents to a minimum. So our announcement to them about wanting to become parents was received as the last nail in the coffin. Clearly if I have a baby with Marilyn, there's little possibility that I'll 'come to my senses.'"

"Most of the members of our families received our news with good wishes. But one of my sisters and one of hers both waited a few months and then raised their issue: what are they supposed to tell their children about how our baby is being conceived? My guess is that they'll wait until the conception has occurred, just to avoid the awkwardness of it with our nieces and nephews. Sarah and I agree it isn't our problem, but we're trying to figure out whether this is a genuine request for help or whether it is a message that, once again, we're the black sheep in the family."

"One of my sisters has been going through infertility treatment for the past year. Her reaction was mixed. On the one hand she was glad to know that someone else in the family was having to work at conceiving a pregnancy; on the other hand, it seems to me that if I conceive before she does it will remind her of her reproductive failure. But now I'm worried that our efforts to get pregnant may take on a competitive edge in her mind. One thought I've had is to send her some of the lesbian literature that frames efforts at conception away from reproductive failure and toward the positive wish to bring a child into the world. I love my sister dearly and would hate for my pregnancy to drive us apart."

Families are important during any developmental stage, but there is a special poignancy when everyone is poised, waiting for the announcement of a much-wanted pregnancy. Lesbian partners already have had ample experience with their families' reactions to their sexual orientation. And, yet, families have many members, each of whom may have a unique relationship with its lesbian siblings, offspring, nieces, aunts, or cousins. So lesbian partners, always trying to anticipate family reactions, probably will not be taken by surprise as they share with relatives their hopes for a baby. But negative reactions are sure to take a toll on them as they decide whom to tell, how to ask for support, and as they answer awkwardly posed questions from various family members. So not only do they bear the suspense of whether or not their method of conception will be successful, they also may endure family lack of emotional support at the very time it would be most appreciated. Many lesbians find comfort in creating their own non-kin families, chosen out of love and compassion, who can be counted on for strong and solid validation.

The non-birthing partner says: "Although we arrived together at the decision of who would try first to get pregnant, I'm worried that while she's learning how to nurse I'll have to be preoccupied with the legalities of adoption."

The birthing partners say:

"Both of us are unhappy and angry that the legal system makes it so complex for a baby to be recognized as having two lesbian parents. It feels intrusive to have to pay for and to go through a home study and all of the legal paperwork associated with an adoption, when both of us know that this baby will be *ours*.

It's partly the cost, it's partly the assumption that we can't be committed parents without a legal document for one of us, and it's very much the legal intrusion on our time and energy just when we're bonding as a family."

"The adoption aggravates both of us. Not only would it be unnecessary if we were a married heterosexual couple, but it sends a message that the non-birthing parent can't be committed to parenthood unless there are legal documents. Of course we're seeking the legal documents so that if, heaven forbid, something terrible should happen to me, Jenna would retain custody of our child. But it's an extra cost, an extra set of appointments on the calendar, and a very real reminder that there's an imbalance in our entitlement to parenthood unless the legal system is involved."

Certainly at the very time a couple is involved in Lamaze classes, furnishing the nursery, making more frequent pre-natal visits, deciding on possible names, and contemplating the changes that a baby will bring in their lives, the prospect of a home study and a legal adoption feels very out-of-place. And this is one of those issues that will not go away. Even if you are legally married and therefore should not need to adopt a child born from this marriage, you probably will go through with the adoption, just to be on the safe side. Depending on what region of the country you may be traveling in, even an adoption may not be recognized as valid, so same sex couples are in a real double bind: damned if they do (because it feels so wrong to have to adopt the child you know to be *yours*), and damned if you don't (in case you're caught in legal limbo somewhere and your parentage is called into question). So the frustration of adopting must be taken in stride with the joy of a new baby in the family.

Therapeutic Tips

The challenge you face as a couple is to accept that your difficulty in conceiving places a unique stress on your relationship. It isn't a stress easily shared with others, because of the privacy many people place around personal issues like sex and reproduction. It isn't a stress that health-care providers are likely to ask about. It isn't a stress that parents or siblings are likely to understand. And it isn't a stress that you and your partner ever anticipated or experienced before.

However, as time moves forward, frustrations mount, schedules are disrupted, and savings accounts are depleted, it is normal and expectable for your emotional resilience to wear thin. Your challenge is not only hoping and planning for parenthood; it is also knowing how to keep your relationship in enough balance so you as a couple can empathize with one another and move forward on a common path. This may be new territory for you, so don't be shy about seeking out resources that can offer new coping skills, open up channels of communication, and bolster your emotional resilience. Here are a few ways you can find additional support:

- Join a support group so that you feel less isolated socially and better connected to couples whose experiences may mirror yours.

- Inquire about whether your infertility clinic provides a therapist with whom you and your partner can discuss the impact of infertility on your relationship. Also inquire whether the clinic provides a support group for couples.

- Become a member of the Infertility Awareness Association of Canada (IAAC) or RESOLVE (the national US infertility association) and learn how other couples address the challenges you and your partner are facing.

- Use Internet chat rooms and resources suggested by IAAC or RESOLVE to find creative resolutions to managing anger and sadness.

- Seek out a therapist who has expertise in couple therapy so the channels of communication with your partner can be rejuvenated and you can feel less stuck.

- Keep some boundaries around your sadness and your frustrations. Agree with your partner on setting time limits on regular discussions about conceiving.

- Weigh the option of taking a vacation from infertility treatment, both to get a rest from the side effects of hormone treatments and to assess with your partner what next steps you are ready to consider.

Four

The Waiting Game: *When Life Is on Hold*

Treating infertility is a time-consuming process, and it is predictable that you will feel as if your life is being held hostage. More than likely you and your partner will be subjected to a variety of medical tests and possibly medical interventions. You may need to take pills, have injections, monitor hormone levels, have surgery, and recover from that surgery. You will spend a lot of time waiting, all the while unable to move forward in your career, take on new challenges, or build up your financial security because of the possible high cost of treatments.

This is a time when many women feel helpless, swept along by the tests and procedures, and as the months progress, far from confident that they will get pregnant. This also is a time when you, like many women, feel dependent on your health-care providers. You find that you wince at impersonal communications, grind your teeth at unreturned telephone calls, and silently chafe at the inflexibility of the scheduling process that rules your life. But because you are so dependent on the medical staff, it feels too risky to vent your feelings. Your life is moving at a sluggish pace, with the tantalizing hope of pregnancy dangling just out of reach.

Feeling stuck, whether by infertility itself, or by others in your life who are unable to support your decisions, can be discouraging and exhausting. As the women in this chapter relate, infertility has catapulted them into a morass of decisions they never envisioned when they first began their efforts to conceive. Most people find that if they can agree on how to proceed, the opinions of employers, parents, in-laws, and other loved ones matter less. Further, most women can find role models in their new communities of infertile women and couples. Support groups, clinic waiting-room conversations, counselors, friends of friends, and chat rooms are all resources that women may want to consult as they try to get "unstuck" and open new doors.

And especially as you experience the frustrations of infertility, you will want to find ways to lift your spirits, distract yourself from disappointing news, consider new options, and nurture your relationships. Finding balance in your life becomes more of a conscious effort now that you are in the midst of medical procedures. Remember that just as you are spending considerable energy engaged in medical treatment, you can soothe some of this stress by identifying and connecting with personal and community resources.

Waiting

Once you begin diagnosis and treatment, there is an initial hopefulness that you're on a new path with pregnancy as a hoped-for outcome. But, as the remarks of the women in this chapter reveal, that hopefulness begins to fade as time marches on and still no pregnancy occurs. Impatience, frustration, sadness, and dependence on health-care providers are familiar responses as month after month pass, with your calendar and your bank account constantly adjusting to clinic procedures. It isn't unusual to feel "stuck," and some couples use this treatment time as an opportunity to seek counseling, both for their own peace of mind and also to open the door a crack to consider other options they might be willing to pursue:

"Once we began to be seen at the clinic, I felt as if the treatment regimen was so much more organized than what I had experienced with my local physician. But, looking back, I had no idea how the variety of tests and treatments would take up so much time. So we grind along, first doing a certain number of months of one procedure. Then when that doesn't result in a pregnancy, we try another couple months of the next procedure on the list. Getting negative test results each month has felt like nails being pounded into our family coffin. Neither my husband nor I want to go through IVF [in vitro fertilization] if we can avoid it, but we're beginning to run out of options."

"It's getting to the point where I'm afraid to call the lab for results when I'm at work, because if my hormone levels aren't up, then I know this is one more lost month. If I'm at work that means I land in the restroom and have a good cry, and my colleagues only need to see my bloodshot eyes to know the news this month isn't good. But if I wait until I get home, often the clinic is closed and then if I'm lucky there's a message on our answering machine. Sometimes I ask Tom to listen to the voice message because I'm tired of always being the first to hear bad news. I recently counted how many months we've been trying to get pregnant — it's been over 30. My friends and family are holding out hope, but I don't know how much longer I can. I'm reaching the point where Tom and I need to look at where we want to go from here. That way, at least, we could ask ourselves the hard questions we've avoided so far — about whether we should seek out a new clinic or begin to consider adoption or surrogacy."

"One of the worst aspects of having my life divided into 'before treatment' and 'waiting for results' is that my emotions are being badly affected by the medication and the failure to get pregnant. There's no longer even a 'good' time of the month. All the days are colored by the hormones I'm taking, and of course everything comes crashing down when the nurse calls with bad news. I've never been a very patient person, and I do well when I'm in control of my life. So now, I feel both out of control and impatient. But each month is more than just a month without a pregnancy. Each month is time spent, money spent, my body being subjected to medications, and my schedule being turned upside down to accommodate medical appointments. I'm even too exhausted to distract myself with friends, hobbies, or a good book. The magazine articles on trying to conceive always end up with the parents cuddling a darling newborn. When will it be my turn? Haven't I waited long enough? One of my infertile friends is seeing a counselor she thinks is very good and, much as I dread adding yet another appointment to my calendar, I'm beginning to think that some counseling sessions might be my best chance at breaking loose from feeling so trapped."

"When Jack and I were first diagnosed as having infertility problems, an infertile friend of ours gave us a book that had more wisdom than I realized at the time. Dr. Seuss's book *Oh, The*

Places You'll Go! captures the path we have traveled to infertility. Right now we're in the place that the book calls 'The Waiting Place,' where no matter what you do you're still stuck. I've faced frustrations in my life, but I've always felt as if there were new doors I could open. Jack and I aren't ready to consider adoption yet, so here we are, dependent on medical professionals to do the best they can to help me conceive. In my wildest dreams I never imagined this pathway to parenthood."

Not Taking On New Challenges

In addition to feeling stuck waiting for a positive pregnancy test, you may feel unable to move ahead with other aspects of your life: career choices, promotions, further education, or moving. These decisions and others are closely tied to whether or when you will become parents, and it seems difficult to move in new directions until the certainty of parenthood has been made clear. The following stories explore how some women feel about their own inability to move forward:

"Our plan was to have two children, and once they were in school I would go back to university to get my master's in education. An advanced degree would open up better-paying career opportunities and also give me more flexibility to be off during the summer months for family time. If I had known a couple of years ago that I'd be getting treated for infertility for four years, I would have gotten my degree earlier. The way things are going now, I don't dare enroll in a graduate program, because what if I get pregnant? But the longer I stay out of school the less professionally productive I feel. And, frankly, if I don't get pregnant, I don't know whether I want to enter a profession that focuses on working with other people's children."

"Last year my boss said to me that he wanted to groom me to take over the position of someone in the company who is due to retire. That person has a lot of responsibility, works long hours, and has made the company the center of his life. So I explained to my boss that once I have children I doubt that I could commit to the additional hours and the travel schedule that would be expected of me. I said it in the throes of lots of medical procedures that had to be carefully timed, so a part of me was aware that I couldn't meet the challenges of the position if I were still being treated for infertility. So here I am stuck in my current work position, without the joy of a baby to take the monotony out of my life."

"I have the perfect job for a parent — I get summers off, I have good vacation and sick-leave benefits, and I can do some work from home. It's not nearly as stimulating as other jobs I could have, but I took it because I wanted to be able to balance work and family responsibilities. But as the months drag on, I realize that this job isn't good for me *now*. I have very few coworkers, the work is fairly repetitive, and there's no social life at lunchtime or after work. So these days it feels lonely, isolating, and boring, just when I need to have some distractions from the disappointments of my infertility treatment. I know I stay in this job as a way of saying to myself that maybe I *will* be a parent soon. But maybe I need to start listening to Mike when he encourages me to get out of the house with him for a quick morning walk, to meet friends for lunch, or to take that evening cooking class at the community college."

"Last month Janice was offered a transfer to a branch of her company that is in another city. This transfer carried a promotion

with it, and the only reason she didn't take it is that we feel
so fortunate to be in the same city as the infertility clinic
where I'm being treated. If we move, the nearest infertility clinic would be four hours round trip, which would have
been exhausting and disruptive for me. I suppose there may
be other opportunities for her later, but it was hard for both
of us that she had to pass up this promotion because I haven't
become pregnant yet."

"As a single woman, I've had to plan pretty carefully for the support system that I can count on if I'm lucky enough to have a
baby. When my boss offered to pay for my education if I would
work in a distant city after I got my master's degree, she seemed
totally puzzled when I turned her down. I explained that I was
trying to get pregnant, and her response was that she was sure I
could manage my education along with parenthood. Well, perhaps I could, if I'm lucky enough to get pregnant in the next
year or so, but she seemed completely unable to grasp that my
support network is *here*, and I can't very well pick that up and
move it to another city."

Infertility and Your Job

Another aspect of feeling that your life is on hold may occur as
you realize that your work and infertility do not mix. Perhaps
it is the inflexibility of your job, the insensitivity of your coworkers, or that infants and children are an integral part of your
work at a time when you are yearning to nurture a baby in your
own home. The dilemma becomes whether you are prepared
to tough out the months of infertility treatment in a job that
causes you stress, whether you will seek another kind of work, or
whether you will leave the workforce altogether. These women

speak about their challenges of juggling infertility treatment and work, which may be the same as your own:

"Initially my boss was reasonably understanding when I told him that I would need to take some sick time for infertility treatments. But I think he believed it would be only at convenient times. Well, now it seems that no time is convenient. And although I'm legally entitled to take sick time, I don't always know from day to day when I'll be scheduled to go in for procedures, and he is getting less and less accepting of my absences. I know I have the union on my side, but the work environment is getting downright unpleasant. I feel as if infertility treatment has become a second job, and of course I have to give it priority. So, given my boss's negative attitude, I'm trying to decide whether I should look for a new job or if we could afford to use Jack's medical benefits, which aren't as good as mine, and just have me quit work until we know if the infertility treatments are going to be successful."

"I've always been proud to be a child welfare worker, and I know my work has made an important difference in the lives of lots of families. But over the past year I've been feeling more and more anger toward the parents who abuse and neglect their children. I used to be able to appreciate the life circumstances that might cause someone to put a child at risk, and I was good about being able to intervene, to set clear limits, and to advocate for the children involved. Lots of people I worked with were able to turn their lives around and become better parents. Now I am consumed with anger toward these parents who treat helpless children with so little love and concern, and when I encounter abusive situations it's all I can do to resist taking the children home myself! I know that my infertility is what has made me react personally rather than professionally. So now I'm struggling with how to take the focus of my work away from children, at least until I'm successful in becoming a parent myself."

"I'm a midwife. My greatest joy is in working with couples during the woman's pregnancy and then delivering healthy children into this world. But I'm realizing that after five years of being treated for infertility, I am feeling jealous of my patients, envious of their abilities to plan their lives so carefully, and downright weepy when I place a newborn into its parent's arms. I worked my whole adult life to be a great midwife, and now infertility is robbing me of being able to take joy in my work. I'm considering taking a leave of absence — maybe to teach students midwifery, which would be less direct contact with pregnant women and infants. Somehow, I need to find a new path to follow while I'm trying to cope with my infertility."

The Financial Crunch

Before you were faced with infertility, you probably had many financial goals and dreams that you wanted to achieve, such as owning a home, saving for retirement, or taking an exciting vacation. However, now that you have new financial challenges to deal with, you might feel like your financial plans are at a standstill and you're not sure how to organize your funds.

In addition, like many infertile women, you probably have become an expert on how to distract yourself on bad days, nurture yourself, and try new experiences at the very time when the one experience you really want eludes you. And the reality is that it usually costs money to cushion yourself against the pain of infertility. And coping with infertility costs money. So you may be stuck between saving money for future infertility or adoption expenses versus spending it on yourself. Perhaps you can gain insight from the stories of these women who coped creatively with the financial challenges of infertility:

"We've been trying hard to watch our savings, since we've decided to pursue adoption if I don't get pregnant in two years. But we know that two years of infertility treatment can be costly, especially when it involves missing days from work, so we're tucking away every spare dollar and that means no new clothes, no vacations, very few dinners out, and modest gifts on birthdays and holidays. Mack and I decided to begin doing some things that would increase our feeling of togetherness and reduce the stress that infertility is causing. He thought I was being dramatic when I said that I planned to meditate twice a day, but after hearing from me about how I felt more able to cope, he is setting aside time for meditation each day too. We both find that it allows us to move through the stress more constructively. Then, since we have to eat at home more, and neither of us is very handy in the kitchen, we decided to make weekend projects of cooking different ethnic foods. If a dish turns out really well, we celebrate by inviting friends over to share it with us. And, just because it is sometimes hard to face the day, we now get up 30 minutes early and take a quick walk together before we have breakfast and leave for work. It lets us feel connected and gets our blood circulating so we have energy for whatever the day brings. I find it really has helped to focus on low-cost activities that bring us closer together."

"Ron and I love the outdoors, and before infertility became such a concern, we used to take vacations all over the country. Now we just can't afford it, so instead we take camping trips that get us into the wilderness, allow us to appreciate the beauty of nature, and challenge us to handle rain, rodents, and rough terrain. We take pride in being able to economize, and it's actually fun to spend weekends in winter planning camping trips for warmer weather. We're thinking of borrowing some cross-country skis and using that as a way of getting outdoors, while avoiding the expenses that go along with downhill skiing."

"As we try to adopt a frugal lifestyle, the people who are becoming our friends are empty-nesters who are paying for their kids' college expenses. We don't end up worrying about conversation moving in the direction of pregnancies and babies, and these friends in their forties and fifties are pretty mellow and easy to be with. Some of them have been in our community much longer than we have, so they often suggest activities that we hadn't thought about. One of the women volunteers in a local soup kitchen, and when I went with her one evening, I decided that this kind of volunteer work was just what I needed to get my mind off my own sadness. Everything is relative, and although I don't have a baby, at least I have a roof over my head, a partner who loves me, and enough nourishing food each day."

Considering Adoption or Surrogacy

Many couples begin their infertility experience with every confidence that they will conceive and have a healthy birth. Then, the months wear on, savings diminish, and mood swings take a toll on their relationship. Perhaps the couple even experiences a pregnancy loss, and all this causes them to rethink their original expectations. For many couples feeling "stuck" in treatment, it can feel somewhat liberating ultimately to use that time to consider what options they might pursue if the woman does not become pregnant. In some cases, this leads to questions about a life without children. In other cases, it opens discussion on what it would mean to consider adoption or surrogacy. The importance of experiencing pregnancy and birth and the significance of genetic ties to one's child are issues that most couples will evaluate. These discussions often wax and wane, depending upon the feelings of each individual. Raising this possibility with one's extended family also brings up issues, particularly if parents or in-laws have strong negative feelings. At some level, beginning to think about the future in terms of opportunities and options is an ideal antidote for the doldrums of the waiting game.

"Our reaction to adoption when we began our infertility treatments was completely negative. We absolutely believed that having a birth child was the only way to accomplish what was important to us: a pregnancy, a delivery, the experience of nursing, and genetic ties. As our diagnosis became more clear, we learned that we would need to use donor sperm, and I found myself feeling uncomfortable that the baby would be genetically related to me but not to Scott. Then after more months of treatment, I realized my body was going through so much with infertility treatments that I didn't have the enthusiasm I once had for pregnancy, delivery, and nursing. I knew then that I just wanted a baby. The more Scott and I discussed it, the more we agreed that adoption, even with its complexities, was feeling more like a good option for us. We've decided to go to some social functions with adoptive families in our community so that we can get to know parents who made the decision we're thinking of making. We're not ready to give up on infertility treatments just yet, but if we do, I want to be ready to open the next door."

"My uterus is malformed and I'll never be able to carry a pregnancy. I had always assumed that I would build my family through adoption. But the more I'm learning about gestational surrogacy, the more interested I am in pursuing that for a couple of cycles. There's nothing wrong with my eggs, and Dick's sperm also seem to be healthy. We know an attorney who specializes in surrogacy, and consulting her will be important, as I understand legal issues differ depending on what part of North America you live in. My sister has even said she would be thrilled if we would consider having her be our surrogate, which is such a loving offer and also may help with potential legal concerns. Ultimately money will become an issue, but for now both Dick and I think of surrogacy as our first option, and if that doesn't result in a healthy pregnancy, we always could turn to adoption."

"Our parents are conservative in many ways, and of their acquaintances who have adopted children, there seem to have been problems and sadness. Never mind that plenty of their friends with birth children have had their share of regrets — our parents are convinced that adoption is the path to certain misery. So, although we've decided not to rock the boat too much, we are definitely going to adopt. We hope that if we are able to find a healthy child our parents will be able to put aside their apprehensions enough to let this baby get a hold on their hearts!"

"As a single woman, with all these months of infertility treatment providing plenty of time to think about future options, I'm feeling increasingly hopeful about pursuing adoption, but even that is complicated. I'm worried that my lack of a partner may count against me. I've been talking with many of my friends about how they could be an extended family for me once I adopt a baby, and they're very excited at the prospect. Many of them are parents, and they know the time and energy it takes to raise a child. As I've watched them I believe I have a pretty good idea of both the sacrifices and the joys. I've had the chance to meet a few single adoptive moms, and they've been very encouraging, so I hope to take to heart some of their suggestions as I decide whether to end these futile months of treatment and begin to look in earnest at how to begin the adoption process."

Therapeutic Tips

Frustrating as it may be to feel that your life is on hold, the examples in this chapter show that you do have options as to how you handle this stage in the infertility journey. Those women who find their lives consumed by infertility are the ones most likely to feel trapped and miserable. It will take both determination and creativity to shape your life (notice, I didn't say "take control") in new ways and to involve loved ones in this effort. If you are someone who feels best when you are calling the shots, you have learned by now that that approach is likely to result in frustration. To soften your approach, I'd like to encourage you to think about the more flexible response of aiming for resilience — the strength that enables you to keep options open, to explore fully what next steps you feel ready to take, and to decide which loved ones can hold you steady in this process.

You are living through a time you never expected, and charting a journey will be a new learning experience. So what are the common threads of solace in this chapter?

- Honor your feelings, but strive not to be consumed by them. Rather than fighting infertility with clenched teeth, try to *accept* it as a part of your life and to think peacefully about how you can move forward as constructively as possible.

- Identify the specific challenges that are a source of frustration and, even as you acknowledge you may not have control over them, brainstorm with loved ones and professionals about alternatives, next steps, new resources, and sources of comfort.

- Think about what comforts you to cushion the frustrations of infertility. Engage your loved ones, if they are willing, in creative plans that they can enjoy with you.

- Consider building some mindful relaxation into your life. Yoga and meditation are practices that have the potential to open your sensibilities and awareness to new ways of thinking about your life.

- Remember that during a time when you are tempted to focus on yourself, you can choose to focus on others whose needs are compelling and whom you may be able to help. This contributes to your conscious efforts not to let your infertility define or consume you.

Five

Scheduled Sex:
When Making Love Becomes Hard Work

In my years of counseling infertile couples, I have encountered only one heterosexual couple whose sexual relationship did not suffer as a direct result of their infertility. Same sex couples have the luxury of being able to separate lovemaking from baby making, which gives them a distinct advantage in their relationship.

The comfort and connection of making love can help couples put aside the worries of the day and bask in the warmth of their relationship. When infertility intrudes, it not only makes sex seem like a chore, but it often wreaks havoc with sexual self-esteem. It is not unusual for women to feel bodily betrayal and to think of themselves as barren. Their bodies are being poked and prodded more than cherished and admired, and they watch with alarm as treatments cause them to retain fluid and gain weight. Women also see their male partners feign disinterest in lovemaking (which has now begun to feel more like obligatory baby making), experience the inability to have or to sustain an erection, and endure producing semen samples on demand, which can be humiliating. Gradually making love is replaced by a carefully timed sequence that results in command ejaculatory performances at the time of your ovulation.

Infertility and Your Sex Life

Most heterosexual couples don't anticipate the sexual fallout that is associated with infertility. And as the importance of conceiving erodes the eroticism of lovemaking, you are likely to feel that infertility has handed you a "double whammy." Not only do you feel unable to conceive without medical intervention, but now it even seems as if your infertility specialist is perched on the bedpost overseeing your most intimate moments. Perhaps you can identify with how infertility has intruded into the sexual lives of some of the couples in this chapter:

"We had always enjoyed the excitement and the closeness of our sexual relationship. As soon as we decided to stop birth control, we were careful about having sex just before the time I expected to ovulate. But we certainly didn't restrict our lovemaking to that time of the month. Not for the first year anyway. But once we began a formal infertility workup, it was as if the doctor were right there in bed with us. Somehow, sex became a very medical thing, and in the process of timing our intercourse, we pretty much let go of being spontaneous. Even though we both miss it, talking about it hasn't brought the zest back into our sex lives."

"Once Mike learned that his sperm count was low and the quality of the sperm was poor, he was completely demoralized, and that affected our sex life dramatically. I felt as if I had to take care of both of us, because he just about melted into the woodwork every night. It didn't matter that I told him he has always been a great lover — as far as he was concerned, if he couldn't produce healthy sperm, he was failing as a husband. It's gotten so bad that he has told me he would understand if I wanted a divorce so I could find someone who could give me babies! I keep telling him that I don't think of him as a baby machine, but his self-esteem is shot to hell, and so is our love life."

"We had a whirlwind courtship, and when we were married three months after we met, we decided to try to conceive right away. After all, we were both in our mid-thirties, and we knew the clock was ticking. Well, it's still ticking three years later, and we're beginning to wonder if we ever had a love life. The first six months were very special, because we felt that our lovemaking, in addition to bringing us close sexually, might also produce a baby who would bring us together in new ways as a family. But once we began our infertility workup, the lovemaking felt more and more obligatory, the timing of intercourse felt like an assignment, and we pretty much lost any sense of spontaneity that we'd ever had. I think the really rough thing for both of us is that we haven't had time to enjoy being married without the cloud of infertility hanging over us. It colors everything we do. I worry that the reason Tod doesn't reach out to me sexually is that I'm becoming a different person from the one he fell in love with — both physically and emotionally. In our honeymoon pictures I was thin, energetic, and smiling. I know I'm not that way any more, and I'm afraid that it may just be easier for him to bail out of this marriage than to stick with the miseries and the broken dreams of our infertility."

"You know, it's amazing to me how many people think that infertility means we don't know how to conceive a baby. Half the advice we're getting from well-meaning friends and relatives has to do with frequency of intercourse, positions after intercourse, jockey shorts — you name it, we've heard it. And let me tell you, it's downright embarrassing when the advice comes from my own mother! I know she means well, but it feels as though she's right there in the bedroom orchestrating our lovemaking according to something she's read in her latest health magazine! No wonder Ross and I feel as if our sex life is screwed up — that's what a lot of people are suggesting. So when we do get into bed, we feel an uncertainty. Everyone else seems to know how to go about lovemaking so that a pregnancy results — what's wrong with us?"

"I can't believe how upset I felt last month when I discovered that Matt had masturbated to satisfy himself sexually. After I was finished ranting about his wasted sperm and his thoughtlessness, I settled down to discuss it. His perspective was that it wasn't my fertile time of the month, and he believed I was so focused on conceiving that I wasn't interested in sex unless I was about to ovulate. My perspective was that I am absolutely focused on our having intercourse when our chances of conceiving are best, but that doesn't rule out making love at other times of the month. But Matt is right in saying that I never initiate sex the way I used to before infertility entered our lives. All of my initiating is based on my ovulation kit, and I guess I believed that he would give some signal when he was in the mood. So it's probably a good thing we sat down and talked about it. It made me realize that I'm so tuned in to my ovulation cycle that I've shut out all the memories of the good sex we've had. I really want to recapture some of that again."

"Ron told me that he needed to take a rest from infertility. So we agreed on three months of no treatment, no calendars, no ovulation kits, no semen samples. But I guess I was naïve to think that our sex life might brighten up a bit. Even before our 'vacation' Ron had trouble maintaining an erection, and the last two times he had to produce semen samples, it took him a couple of hours. The humiliation of sex on command has taken a terrible toll on him. So for him, the vacation from infertility also included a vacation from sex — I think he was afraid that his experiences with not being able to have an erection would reappear, and he just wanted to avoid that humiliation. So I'm going to try to encourage him to arouse me without intercourse, and see if maybe we can find new ways of pleasuring each other. What I'm most worried about is that when the three months are over he won't want to end this vacation. The cost of his being sexually humiliated just may be too high."

"Sam and I both work in pretty demanding jobs, and we are each expected to travel a lot. Initially when I didn't get pregnant, we thought that the stress of our lives was to blame. Then, when we took all of our charts to an infertility clinic, they pointed out to us that we were rarely in the same *part of the country* around the time that I ovulated. So before we proceeded with any treatment, we decided to get a grip on our travel and work schedules. We needed to see whether we could be together in bed at the right time of the month! Well, we've managed to minimize our travel for the next six months, but now that we're both at home more, we're entirely focused on having my ovulation cycle determine when we have sex. But we really aren't having much sex at other times. I'm not sure what's going on. It's true we're both exhausted by our work and the late hours, but I'm also sensing that, given how good we are at our jobs, trying to conceive has become another job we're trying to succeed at. And we can't ask our bosses to keep us off the travel circuit for more than half a year, so we're actually under the gun to conceive quickly. But there's a part of me that would like to step off the fast track so that our lives together can include more sexual closeness, even when it has nothing to do with conception."

"We don't feel entitled to enjoy sex for its own sake, not when we're such miserable failures at conceiving. So our sexual encounters are programmed by the calendar, pretty mechanical, and tied to baby making. The more I think about it, it's not just sex that we don't feel entitled to enjoy. We've pretty much given up everything that was fun in the early years of our marriage. Either it costs too much, or it's too much trouble, or it gets in the way of treatments, or it requires a commitment we don't feel we can make until we know whether or not we're going to be able to have a baby. So we get up each morning, go to work, come home, read or watch TV, and go to bed, and it begins again the next morning. My mother says she thinks we should get counseling because we both seem so depressed, and maybe she's right. It's one thing not to be able to have a baby, but it's another to watch your relationship go down the tubes in the process."

"Stew and I are so blessed to have Amy, who was born five years ago. But in some ways secondary infertility feels especially unfair. Here we are, knowing that we've successfully conceived once. And no one can pinpoint what the problem is. In the meantime, here is Amy, who knows that I go to the doctor for help in getting pregnant, asking when a new brother or sister is going to be born. I think Stew and I want this baby as much for her as we do for ourselves. We find ourselves becoming absorbed with Amy, and each night we fall into bed too tired to make love, except when my ovulation kit tells us that the time is right. Our lives are so busy that we don't set a priority on making time for sex that isn't aimed at conception. Parenthood is very special for us, but there are times that I think we need to pay attention to ourselves as lovers, not just as parents."

"I've had two miscarriages, and there's a part of me that is afraid to get pregnant again because I don't know if I can stand the heartbreak of losing another pregnancy. And Aaron has pretty much told me that he feels guilty, because he's the one who made me pregnant. So here we are in this awful dilemma: we want to conceive, but we're terrified of another miscarriage. Of course this has taken an awful toll on our sex life, since we associate pregnancy loss as an outcome of lovemaking."

"So many infertile people I know say that their lovemaking has been shot to hell. But once Bob and I found out that medical procedures are the only way I'll be able to conceive, we were able to separate having sex from making babies. Now we know that if we have sex, it is for the pure fun and lust of it all. We pretty much avoid sex after each medical procedure, because we're afraid of disrupting the embryo from implanting in my uterus, but when the test results come back negative and we've come to terms with one more disappointment, we know we're in the clear for a few more weeks to enjoy each other sexually. When we were first diagnosed with infertility, I told Bob that we would have to work really hard not to let this stress take a toll on our marriage. And for both of us, the joy and the comfort of lovemaking have helped sustain us through the past couple of years. Much as I hate being dependent on doctors to help us get pregnant, it's a blessing that we haven't lost our sex lives to infertility."

Seeking Counseling for Your Sex Life

There's little question that lovemaking is likely to be a casualty of your infertility struggle, unless you are a lesbian or unless you know that intercourse will not produce a pregnancy. One's sex life is often too awkward to discuss in a support group, too "non-medical" to discuss with your physician, and too personal to discuss with friends and family. Counselors can help individuals and couples think through ways to keep the sexual flame alive despite the onslaught of infertility or pregnancy loss.

If you find your sex life dwindling in the midst of the many stresses of infertility, this is an ideal time to consider meeting with a counselor to discuss ways of separating the hard work of baby making from the comfort and satisfaction of lovemaking. If you are using the services of an infertility clinic, inquire about whether a social worker or a psychologist is on staff. If not, the Infertility Awareness Association of Canada (IAAC) or RESOLVE can provide the name of the nearest support group, which will likely have a referral list of counselors who specialize in working with infertile couples and individuals. Or, if there is no support group in your area, you may be able to find support from the social worker of your local hospital, a family service society in your area, or any infertile acquaintances who may themselves have had a good experience with a counselor. Some counselors have a sliding fee scale, so don't let money stand in the way of getting help. Above all, don't give up lovemaking; it is too precious to lose. With some effort, you can find a caring professional who will help you sort out the important sexual issues in your struggle with infertility, such as the couple in this story has done:

"Our counselor asked about our sex life on the first visit! I was shocked speechless, but she laughed and said that sexual spontaneity was an expected casualty of infertility, and that we'd probably feel better knowing that. Ethan and I hadn't even talked about it to each other, so it was pretty awkward having this conversation with an absolute stranger. But, to our surprise, she offered some advice and some ideas that we've followed, and our sex life has rebounded somewhat. Don't get me wrong — I still have no interest in sex when a bad test result comes back, and I don't always tell Ethan when my period is over because sometimes I'd rather be held than be sexual, but at least we're not as remote from each other sexually as we were before counseling. Our counselor has suggested that we save the bedroom for lovemaking and for sleeping — no reading, no computers, no TV, no eating, and especially no talking about problems, including infertility. Her theory is that if we have distractions or unpleasant associations with what we do in the bedroom, it will be harder to associate that room with sexuality, with desire, and with closeness. She also suggested that we have some fun with our sex life — candles, massages, suggestive lingerie, erotic magazines. Now, I have to admit, some of the things she suggested we hadn't even thought about *before* we were infertile! But it's been a kick seeing what new ideas we can come up with. And Ethan and I agreed that one week he would initiate sex at least one time, and the next I would. We're in a much better place with our sex lives than before we began counseling. We still feel the emptiness of not having a baby, but at least we have the kind of sexual closeness that means so much."

Therapeutic Tips

In earlier chapters I've emphasized the importance of taking care of yourself as you deal with the stress caused by infertility diagnosis and treatment. In this chapter I have looked at sexual distancing as an especially unwelcome price that you pay while you try to conceive. And, at the risk of sounding like a broken record, I will gently remind you that taking care of yourself and your relationship must include careful attention to your love life. Why is it especially vulnerable? It takes time when you have no time; it takes energy when yours is waning or depleted; it takes initiative when your focus is on following doctors' orders; it takes self-esteem when yours may be low; and it takes a joyful anticipation when you feel the only source of joy would be a baby in your arms.

Now that you understand the psychological factors that can contribute to the sexual distance you're experiencing, here are some suggestions for lighting a fire (or at least a warm glow!) in your love life:

- Talk to your partner about the changes in your sexual intimacy since you began trying to conceive. Use this conversation as a way of blaming infertility for your lack of sexual spontaneity. Affirm how erotic you still find your partner; how much you cherish the closeness, comfort, and joy of good sex; and how you want to think of ways to recapture and reinvigorate your love life.

- Once you are openly communicating about your wish to welcome lovemaking back into your lives, see if you can pinpoint the deterrents and figure out how to work around them. Some of the examples in this chapter may give you ideas of how other couples have given their sex lives a jump start, and you'll undoubtedly be able to build on those ideas for your own relationship.

- Be kind to yourselves. Start out slowly, celebrate small sexual pleasures, and don't be deterred by inevitable missteps and disappointments. Keep the lines of communication open so you stay on the same page about what brings you joy and what you need to rethink. Be sure to give positive feedback to each other.

- Experiment with new sexual strategies. Rent DVDs, read books, buy some sexy lingerie — and remember that this is not a scientific experiment! Laugh, be tender, be goofy, be loving. There's always time to create sexual closeness.

- And remember: no pressure! Sexual expression needn't involve intercourse if this reminds you too much of baby making. You can even forget orgasms if you're not in the mood. Kissing, licking, caressing, snuggling, touching — the list of ways you can pleasure one another to reaffirm your sexual joy is endless. Don't wait!

Six

Celebrations and Special Events:
Coping with Gatherings

There's no question that infertility alters your perspective on life. Now more than ever, your attention is devoted to your body, your doctors, your medical procedures, your test results, and your hypothetical future plans. Scheduling medical appointments and procedures around work and other obligations requires a fine-tuned sense of organization, as well as patience, politeness, and cooperation.

And then, all of a sudden, you find yourself thrown off balance by an invitation to a baby shower, a christening, a family holiday celebration, or any event filled with children. You and your partner find it hard enough to be celebratory these days, but when such events are focused on children, the pain is even more acute. What to do? This chapter explores various situations that you may encounter and how some women have chosen to deal with them.

Baby Showers

Baby showers are probably one of the most difficult events you may be asked to attend. In this case, the entire focus of the party is on the expectant mother and her baby, which is exactly the position you want to be in but can't. Here are a few stories that may resonate with your own experiences:

"You know, I haven't told many people that Jason and I have been trying for two years to conceive. So, as far as our friends are concerned, we've just decided not to begin our family yet. The last few baby showers I managed to drag myself to were filled with comments like 'You shouldn't wait too much longer at your age,' and 'Surely you can hear your biological clock ticking by now!' and 'What are you waiting for?' It's nobody's business but ours whether or when we decide to have children, but now that we have been trying so hard, these remarks really sting. Since I'm such a private person and I'm not ready to be open about our infertility, I've just decided to decline invitations to showers."

"The baby shower bit is pretty painful to attend, but shopping for a gift is what's really hard for me. Here I'm standing in a store devoted to darling little outfits, fun little toys, and books for babies and toddlers, and all I can think is 'I want to buy these for *my* baby! Why does it always have to be someone else's baby getting these cute presents?' Finally, one day I just decided to buy a whole huge bunch of baby books. That way whenever I get a baby shower invitation or a birth announcement I'll never have to step foot into a baby store again. Books are fine for boys or girls, and if I'm lucky enough to have a baby of my own, we'll already have started the library!"

"I'm finished with baby showers. It's bad enough that they come at the end of eight or nine months of ultrasound pictures, swollen bellies, swollen ankles, maternity outfits, and mounting excitement. What's worse is that women at the shower just assume that this happy event for the mother-to-be strikes a responsive chord for everybody — not for me. Enough is enough. I know I can find enough 'previous commitments' to get out of attending. My real challenge is how to avoid all the excitement when the baby is actually born and brought into the office to be admired. Disappearing for a couple of hours at a time will take some real creativity on my part, but I think I'm up to that challenge too."

"It seems as if my entire circle of girlfriends is pregnant. And, what's worse, some of these pregnancies are not even planned. So with four close friends whose bellies are starting to swell, I finally decided to be clear about our infertility. One afternoon when we were all together, I just blurted it out. I told them that, although I was happy for them, I just ached inside that I couldn't be pregnant too. I said that the doctors don't know what the problem is, and that it could take a long time to go through all the tests and procedures available, and even then I might not get pregnant. I told them I didn't want my infertility to put a wedge between us at a time that they are so involved in getting ready for their babies, but that I would really appreciate if they wouldn't talk about their pregnancies when I'm around. I told them not to invite me to their baby showers. And I told them that the most painful thing of all for me right now is to be around little babies, so please not to expect me to visit after their baby is born. You could have heard a pin drop. I had tears in my eyes and so did they as they gave me big hugs and told me they had no idea I was going through such a struggle.

We talked a lot that day, as I told them that I knew this would be a challenge to our friendship. But, after all the conversation died down, we agreed that they could get together for baby-and-mom events without me feeling rejected, and those who are already moms said they know they will welcome the chance to get out and not talk about parenthood after the baby is born. Frankly, I feel lucky to have such good friends. I don't know how things will play out, but at least I raised the subject, I told them what I needed from them, and I can always go back to that if they forget and start to wax poetic about their infants when I'm around."

Religious Rituals

The religious rituals associated with infants may vary, but their effect on infertile women is often predictable. Here is an event with the focus on a darling little one, with proud parents, grand-parents, and other family members gathered in a house of worship for a familiar ritual. Except that you find yourself wishing to be anywhere but focusing on this adorable baby who brings you sadness in the midst of everyone else's happiness. Able as you might have been to remove yourself from pregnant friends and their newborns, the family expectations for your attendance at a religious ritual are often not easy to negotiate. And, to make it worse, this ritual may have been preceded by the request that you be the godmother of this child, and your need to decline that request. You may find that you identify with the emotions of the women in this chapter who feel trapped by their loved ones' expectations:

"When my brother and his wife asked my husband and me to be the godparents of their baby, I know they were confused by our silence and our request to talk it over. Although they knew about our infertility, it turns out that they thought the next best thing would be for us to have a godchild. Well, maybe that would work for some people, but for my husband and me, being godparents would just be a constant reminder of the baby we may never have. Both of us had agreed even before my brother's invitation that we would keep our distance from that baby for the first year or two, and then see how painful it was to be around it. So we thanked them for the honor of the invitation and explained that we just weren't emotionally ready to become close to a baby when we couldn't have one of our own. I don't think that my brother and his wife 'got it,' but at least they weren't offended, and fortunately I come from a large family so there are lots of other siblings he can approach."

"I agreed to be my best friend's baby's godmother when both of us were a few months pregnant. Susan and I had both learned we were pregnant with girls, and we had so much fun wondering if they would grow up to be best friends too. Then, at four months, I had a miscarriage; I was devastated. Of course she came right over to the house when I came home from the hospital. We talked and we cried, because it was a loss that touched both of us. A few weeks later I realized that I could not be her baby's godmother. I knew that Susan's daughter would forever remind me of the baby I lost, and the pain would just be too great if I were her godmother. When I told this to Susan, it was as if she had anticipated my decision — it just shows how well she knows me. And, bless her heart, she told me not to give it another thought, that the important thing is that she and I will always be close, and that it will be up to me to decide how her baby will fit into my life."

"Christenings are a big thing in our family. They're not just religious occasions, they're an excuse for a family reunion, a chance for the siblings in the family to get together, and an opportunity for the grandparents to admire their brood. Since most of my siblings live nearby, and even those who live far away fly to town when their babies are to be christened, we see christenings as special family rituals. So with that as a backdrop, imagine my family's reaction when Bruce and I explained that we wouldn't be in town for the next christening. We've been struggling with infertility for five years, and in that time the four christenings we've attended have been progressively more painful. We resent that God hasn't blessed us with a baby, we have no interest in doting on any more family newborns, and I always feel as if I'm in a field of fertile rabbits when I'm around my sisters and sisters-in-law. Needless to say, my parents were floored. The family grapevine began to operate instantly, so I quickly got on the phone to my sister whose baby was to be christened and explained that I was happy for her baby's healthy birth, but being infertile has made both Bruce and me very sad around newborns. She said that she wished we would change our minds, and I said it would only increase our feelings of unhappiness to come to the christening when our hearts were aching. I explained that this had to do with taking care of ourselves at a stressful time, and that in no way did I want to take away from her joy of being a new mother. I think it helped to be direct about it, but it was one of the most difficult conversations I've ever had."

"I was raised in a Catholic family. So the Church was a big issue when I came out as a lesbian and had a commitment ceremony joining me to Janet five years later. My parents attended the ceremony reluctantly, more because they didn't want to lose me than because they accepted Janet into our family. So now that I'm going through donor insemination, my parents are raising the importance of having the baby baptized. Frankly, since I've been trying unsuccessfully to get pregnant for six months, I have no interest in a baptism. Especially a baptism in the Catholic Church, where being a lesbian is tons worse than being a lapsed Catholic. But this is going to be a big deal with my parents, who probably want to protect the baby against our 'lifestyle' and think that a baptism is a good start in that direction."

"After my sister had a baby boy, the bris was scheduled at the temple and Jacob and I were expected to attend. I had concentrated so much on how I could minimize contact with this new baby that I'd completely forgotten about the bris, where everyone would be celebrating my nephew's healthy birth. I didn't have the courage to absent myself from the bris itself, but Jacob and I sat way in the back of the temple, and we left as soon as we could. I know my mother felt we were being rude, and I suspect my sister did too, but I thought we fulfilled my family obligation by being there at all. I've resolved that if anyone in the family makes so much as a reference to our brief participation, I'll remind them that our infertility feels like an open wound when we're around babies, and we did the best we could to honor our new nephew while still taking care of ourselves."

Holidays

Holidays are times that families come together. They are times that people celebrate. And they are often symbolically linked with hopefulness, thanksgiving, and parenthood, none of which will be high on your list of topics close to your heart. To make the holidays even more toxic, this often is a time when the family gathering focuses on infants or young children, and where various relatives will be pregnant or nursing. We all know that holidays, joyful as they are expected to be, can be a source of stress for anyone trying to meet high expectations of these family events. But infertility introduces an additional stress for you if you are trying to keep your distance from babies and pregnant relatives. So see whether any of these scenarios strike a responsive chord (and make a mental note of some the creative solutions proposed for holiday dilemmas):

"Thanksgiving is one of the toughest holidays for Jim and me. The family tradition is to gather at his parents' house, and usually about 20 people are there. For sure at least one person will be pregnant or nursing, and there are always a handful of little kids. So on top of having to celebrate a holiday when I can't think of much to be thankful for, I'm besieged with fertility at every turn. Jim's mom is a dear, and she has been very concerned about us. So Jim and I decided that we would offer to come to the house early in the day and give her lots of help getting the turkey in the oven, getting the table set, bringing over extra chairs, and just having some time to talk to her and his dad without the whole family around. But we told his parents that after the meal, instead of hanging around watching the little kids and listening to his siblings talk about parent-stuff, we would help with the dishes and then leave early to have some quiet time for ourselves. And we explained why. Luckily for us, they understood. And in some ways I think our plan allows them to dote on the grandchildren without feeling hampered by our presence. This arrangement doesn't do anything to help me feel more thankful, but at least I'm not subjecting myself to an unnecessarily lengthy family get-together."

"The holiday I hate most is Mother's Day. For the longest time I was able to see that as a day when my siblings and I sent cards to our mother. Then as my sisters and girlfriends had babies, Mother's Day began to be a day celebrated by my own generation. And I was still able to keep the focus on my mother, so that was okay. But last Mother's Day in church I was floored when a person holding corsages asked if I were a mother. I said no, and the person nodded and didn't give me a corsage. Then it dawned on me that mothers were entitled to corsages and non-mothers weren't! But it got worse. The minister actually asked all mothers to stand up at one point in the service so that the congregation could pay special tribute to them. At that point I just lost it. I left the church in tears, with Allan close behind me. When I got home and got a grip on myself, I wrote the minister a letter explaining the pain that I had experienced that day in church as someone who wanted more than anything to be a mother. I explained that there were probably others in the congregation whose hearts were aching because of infertility, pregnancy loss, or the death of a child. And I ended by asking that he not make a special tribute to mothers on Mother's Day, since there are many non-mothers in the congregation who love children and who contribute to the lives of children. To my great satisfaction, he telephoned me at home to thank me. He apologized for having been so shortsighted, and he asked my permission to share my letter, anonymously, with a group of local religious leaders whom he thought could learn from what I had written. So out of my misery did come some good, but I wonder how many other non-mothers have vowed never to go to church on Mother's Day again?"

"This year for Christmas, Art and I have decided to take a trip to the Caribbean. I know my entire family will be shocked that we're skipping the celebration, but honestly, each year is getting more painful than the last. My siblings are producing more and more babies, and I'm increasingly stressed out at the sight of the kids opening up their presents and their stockings with adults smiling all around. In my family, Christmas is really focused on the children, which is fine for the kids and their parents, but what about us? Where do we fit in, with no pregnancy for six years, no baby after two miscarriages, and no prospect of becoming parents by Christmas? So this year we'll try something new and see if we can have a soothing and relaxing time away from the reminders of parenthood and Santa Claus."

"You know the holiday that bums me out the most? Halloween! Can you believe it? But when I was a kid that was my favorite holiday, and even now the joy of kids getting ready to trick-or-treat can be heard up and down our block. Before we had to deal with infertility, we would decorate our front porch, and I'd get into a wacky costume. But I think this year we'll either hire a neighborhood teenager to answer the door or we'll just darken all our lights and leave town for the evening. It just makes me too sad to see so many little kids when I can't dress up any trick-or-treaters in my family!"

"Making New Year's resolutions has been a miserable challenge ever since we were diagnosed with infertility. It's bad enough that another year has passed without a baby to share our lives. The thought that I should focus on changing or improving something about myself is downright infuriating. Just getting through the year in one piece is an ordeal in itself. I was about at the point of chucking the idea of New Year's resolutions altogether when another infertile friend told me about how she approaches the New Year. She makes a commitment to do something for others — whether it's a little volunteer work each month, a good deed for an elderly neighbor, a financial contribution to a worthy cause . . . As she says, infertility is such a self-absorbing phenomenon that unselfish acts help her to focus on the needs of others. That works for me much better than anything that reeks of self-improvement."

"Hanukkah is a holiday that always has been lots of fun in our family. When we were little, my brothers and I felt lucky to be Jewish at a time of the year when we would be getting gifts for eight nights and our Christian friends only had Christmas as their gift-giving day. Anyway, now the shoe is on the other foot, as I've been sending gifts to my nieces and nephews year after year, wishing that I had a baby whose eyes would light up at the sight of the menorah candles. So this year I decided that rather than brave the holiday-shopping maze, with all the stressed-out parents and excited children, I would send checks to my nieces and nephews and let them each choose one gift that they know is from Jeff and me. We quietly celebrate Hanukkah at home with potato latkes and lighting the menorah, but the focus is much more on our being together as a couple than it is on making a big production of presents for the children in our extended family."

Family Celebrations

Whether the family is just you and your partner, or it extends to other relatives, there are traditions that everyone assumes you will continue to celebrate, even as your infertility is causing you to re-evaluate whether you want to. How to communicate with family about your different plans "this year," or how to regroup and celebrate in a new way, may be challenges you are contemplating. Perhaps these scenarios will sound familiar:

"My brother and his wife invite the whole family for their kids' birthday parties. That usually adds up to about 12 people, most of whom are kids. It's pretty chaotic, not at all relaxing, and increasingly painful as we feel the sadness of being infertile. So this year we told my brother and sister-in-law that being around that many children was just too much of a reminder of the family life we yearned for. We said that we'd stop by before the party to drop off our gift and give the birthday child a hug, but we wouldn't stay for the party. They seemed surprised, and I really think it never occurred to them that being around children is hard for us. Our plan worked just fine, and we expect we'll continue this way until we have some birthday celebrations that we can invite the cousins to attend."

"Early in our marriage our anniversary was a time that we tried to get away from work for a long weekend together. But the last couple of years we didn't make much of an effort, because one year our anniversary coincided with an infertility procedure, another year I got my period and was so depressed I cancelled our plans. When I mentioned this to the counselor I've been seeing, she reminded me that even when our greatest hopes are denied, we still have choices. She meant that even while we're still not able to have a baby, we can still make choices about creating positive experiences for ourselves. So Sean and I have decided that we'll time our anniversary celebration so it won't conflict with either my ovulation or my period — is that crazy or what? And we've vowed not to raise the topic of our infertility or future options — just to enjoy the anniversary time for what it is. With both of us concentrating on making this a special time together, perhaps it will bring some of the comfort back into our marriage after all the stress."

"My birthday is getting harder and harder to bear. When I was 28 and trying to get pregnant, having a birthday just seemed like another year had gone by. But now that I'm 36, not only have *lots* of years gone by, but with each one I'm losing the likelihood of being able to conceive. So each birthday is now a bitter reminder of diminishing possibilities for a pregnancy. And of course with that perspective, who even wants to celebrate? Not me. I've told everyone in the family that birthdays aren't happy occasions for me, but I've also made some suggestions for those family members who want to give me a gift. Some of them have arranged to send me a lovely bouquet twice a month; another family member knows how much I love fresh oranges and grapefruit in the winter, so she sends me a huge citrus carton every January; and a dear friend who lives in New York uses her frequent-flier miles to send me an airline ticket for a long weekend every spring, and we have a lovely time together. Spreading out my birthday gifts over the year is so much better than being reminded on my birthday that I'm a year older."

Dealing with Gatherings on Your Own Terms

Holidays and family celebrations are emotionally loaded, even without infertility as a backdrop. Since so many family events focus on children, you will need to decide whether the familiar and traditional ways of celebrating continue to bring you pleasure. If not, remember that no one should make you feel compelled to participate in events that are stressful.

Often friends and family believe that holidays and family celebrations are a cushion against the stresses of life, that rituals are comforting, and that children are a reminder of the future of the family. But in truth, celebrations often have expectations associated with them that are too difficult to fill. The stress of a holiday season can leave the celebrants more exhausted than exhilarated, and the large gathering of family members often precludes any meaningful one-on-one conversations. Individuals trying to conceive are not alone in feeling shortchanged and short-tempered at holiday time; however, at least you are more clear than most about the source of your lingering sadness. That knowledge can empower you to make constructive changes in the familiar rituals that have acquired sharp edges.

In addition, you can choose to take the opportunity to enlighten friends and family members about your reasons for changing your participation in celebrations. Infertility is not an invisible force in your life, and your loved ones need to know that you are working hard to make constructive decisions. You will want to emphasize that your decision has to do with taking care of yourself at a difficult time and you are not upset with them in any way. Even though the effect of your decision is to change familiar rituals, you need to ask your friends and family to be understanding and supportive.

Therapeutic Tips

We begin by assuming that because your loved ones believe family traditions are joyful, they are blind to the pain they may cause for you. Your loved ones look forward to rituals as the glue that holds the family together; you, on the other hand, know that some of these rituals are an increasing source of alienation and sadness as you yearn for motherhood.

So it's time to clarify your needs around how to avoid or redefine painful rituals; it's time to be clear with loved ones about your new decisions; it's time to emphasize that your focus is on taking care of yourself; and it's time, hopefully, to express to loved ones how they can be supportive and how much you appreciate their understanding:

- Suggest new family rituals.

- Redefine the ways in which you participate in seasonal celebrations.

- Include your infertile friends in your lives at times of the year that are filled with children.

- Focus on yourself and your partner as a family in your own right — stop trying to "fit in" to celebrations and instead define your own form of celebration.

- Emphasize the enduring love that you and your partner share, your readiness to honor both sadness and joy, and your commitment to those friends and family members who understand how infertility is shaping your life.

- Above all, be kind to yourself. Learn what leisure activities you enjoy most, what friends and relatives are most understanding, and what new rituals bring you the most comfort — and then indulge yourself!

Seven

Another Shoulder to Lean On:
Support Groups and Therapists

You have learned that your life is being redefined by your infertility. It affects your relationships, your finances, your body, your mental health, and your future life choices. Some days your infertility is bearable and other days it is simply overwhelming. The earlier chapters in this book cover many of the stresses you are trying to cope with, but there are some infertility issues that will make you feel so vulnerable that you wish you had another shoulder to lean on. Since your partner, friends, and family have provided their shoulders already, and you may not want to lean on them too much, you may decide to seek support elsewhere.

Chapter 1 introduced support groups and therapists as additional "shoulders," those people in your community who are committed to helping you feel more empowered. (Different counseling professionals may refer to themselves as "therapists" or as "counselors," so I will use these terms interchangeably.) This chapter will go into more detail about how to decide what source of emotional support would be most helpful for you and maybe also for your partner; how you can locate a support group that is a good fit with your needs; how to find a therapist; and what to expect from counseling sessions. It can feel like a daunting prospect but, as you will learn from the voices in this chapter, other people can open up new perspectives on your infertility, provide creative ways of coping, offer information about additional resources, and move you away from a preoccupation with your medical treatment and toward efforts to be more emotionally resilient.

I would like to make a note about the Internet here. Many women enjoy its advantages of being convenient, anonymous, and easy to access. However, it also has disadvantages: it may offer inaccurate information, it may keep you alone at your computer rather than out interacting with people who care about you, and it may prevent you from learning about local resources. So, if you find the Internet helpful, you should continue to use it, but do consider expanding your network to include local support groups and counselors. They can best help track your ups and downs over time and help you when you are especially vulnerable.

In-Clinic Support Groups

Some infertility clinics provide support groups for patients who are undergoing infertility treatment, although, given the distance that many people have to travel, the membership of the group may vary from one meeting to the next. Clinics also provide support groups for patients undergoing procedures such as in vitro fertilization (IVF), which give new participants an opportunity to learn from those who have undergone a procedure multiple times.

Also, local hospitals may offer support groups for people who have experienced a pregnancy loss, including miscarriages, ectopic pregnancies, and stillbirths. Such groups usually meet once a month and are facilitated by a mental health professional associated with the hospital. Clinic support groups are likely to be led by an experienced professional who understands group dynamics and who is familiar with clinic procedures and the pressures they put on patients. Read on as women share their experiences attending in-clinic support groups:

"The nurse who led our support group at the infertility clinic was very knowledgeable about IVF, and all the couples attending the group were IVF patients. Some had had as many as five IVF procedures, but many of us were first-timers. It definitely helped to hear the perspectives of the experienced couples. Even though the nurse knew the medical protocols, the other couples were able to address the emotional aspects of IVF that were becoming such a big part of our lives. They knew what IVF represented to us — the last hope for a birth child. They also understood the financial pressures. The experienced couples knew the anguish of waiting for news about hormone levels after IVF, and they were living proof that if IVF fails the first time, you can try again, assuming that you have the money or the insurance coverage. Those clinic support groups were the emotional glue that helped us through a terribly anxious time."

"One aspect of the clinic support group that I found especially helpful was the support to the partners of the women undergoing IVF. In our group we had husbands and male partners. The facilitator knew how to draw the guys into the discussion. She encouraged the group to offer support not only to the women who were being shot full of hormones but also to the guys who had been the stoic rocks for their partners. It helped the guys to feel involved and it also gave them a chance not to be so stoic any more. Most of the men felt apprehensive, since the outcome of the procedure would have such emotional ramifications for their families. The facilitator addressed the issue of temporary impotence caused by the pressure of producing a fresh semen sample on the day of the procedure. Who would have thought that the men would be willing to speak to such an issue? But in our group, *all* the guys were worried about not being able to produce on command. My husband felt the group was a safe and supportive place to go when none of his friends or relatives had a clue what he was going through."

Community Support Groups

Community support groups may have evolved informally among infertile couples hoping to share resources and information. And some communities may have support groups sponsored through the Infertility Awareness Association of Canada (IAAC) or RESOLVE, the national US infertility association. Although some group facilitators may be mental health professionals, many are members of the local community who have a personal history of infertility and who have acquired expertise and empathy by reaching out to newly infertile people.

"When I went to my first support group I was most worried about how much I would be expected to disclose. I'm a pretty private person, and our community is small enough that I expected I might know some of the people who came to the support group. Cliff simply refused to go. So I felt very alone as I walked in the door that first time. There was coffee and a literature table, so I occupied myself with those until someone came up and introduced herself by her first name, which felt comfortable to me. She said that she had been coming to the support group for the past two years, and we talked a little about her situation, but she didn't ask about mine. After more people arrived, the leader asked us all to find seats, and she welcomed us to the group and reminded us of the confidentiality policy that we were expected to observe. She encouraged people to say as much or as little about themselves as they chose to. About eight people were there that evening. A few gave their first names and a brief summary of their infertility situation. I decided just to give my first name and to say that I was there for my first time and that I didn't know any other people in the community who were grappling with infertility. When we finished going around the group, the leader asked if anyone had an issue to raise. One woman had just had a very unpleasant experience with her mother-in-law, who expected her to attend a baby shower for a family member. The group talked about this, and the leader was very good about providing specific examples of how to be clear and assertive about our needs, even when dealing with insensitive people. Several others shared personal examples of ways that they had addressed similar family insensitivities. The rest of the meeting was a general discussion of how to communicate our needs to our partners, since that was apparently a common issue. That first meeting really drew me in without threatening my privacy. As I came to more meetings I felt increasingly able to share, and I was just so touched by the thoughtfulness of the people in the group."

"The time that I was most grateful to be in a support group was during my first year of infertility. I came to a meeting saying that I had an awful pain in my abdomen, and that I was really feeling rotten. One of the members asked if I had told my gynecologist, and I said I had and that his nurse had told me to wait 24 hours and come in tomorrow if it wasn't better. A woman who had had an ectopic pregnancy told me that I shouldn't wait, and she drove me right then to the emergency room. Sure enough, it was an ectopic pregnancy, and I was rushed into surgery. The doctors weren't able to save my tube, but they did save my life. That incident catalyzed our support group into sending a few members to visit my clinic to discuss how to prevent such a close call in the future."

"About six months after I began going to support group meetings, I was hospitalized for surgery to clean out endometrial tissue from my abdominal cavity. Members of the support group had asked if I would like visitors in the hospital and at home. We have no family nearby, so of course I did. Not only did someone from the support group come to visit in the hospital every day, but when I got home group members delivered dinners to us for two weeks. Jerry, who had never gone to any meetings, was so touched by their thoughtfulness that now he attends meetings with me, which has really brought us closer together."

"The woman who leads our community support group has two children she adopted after six years of infertility problems. Our community is small enough that all the gynecologists and urologists in town give her name out to any of their patients who are having trouble conceiving. She is so well known now that people from surrounding towns come to the monthly meetings. We get about seven or eight members each month, and she is very good at drawing people out about the issues they're struggling with. She's been doing this for so long that she knows about all sorts of community resources, from counselors to adoption workers. Many of us have needed to go out of the community for high-tech treatment, and she has even given us names of other people who were willing to share the experiences they've had with certain clinics and hospitals. So, in addition to being a really sensitive support group leader, she has a wealth of information about different options to pursue."

As these stories show, support groups can provide much-needed solace and understanding, as well as information about local and regional resources. However, as I mentioned in Chapter 1, ask beforehand about the group's policy on allowing pregnant women to attend meetings. Those that allow pregnant members recognize that the bonds of the support group are very important to a woman who has achieved a much-wanted pregnancy and who may be fearful of miscarriage. Those that do not allow pregnant women have established this policy because the members have decided that having a pregnant member in their midst would be distracting and emotionally distressing. Whatever the practice of the group, it is likely that much discussion has gone into the decision to adopt the policy.

Counselors and Therapists

As helpful as support groups can be, there also are times that seeing an individual counselor is most appropriate. If you are concerned about privacy, need more personal attention than a group can provide, are overwhelmed by stress, or need special help to think through very personal issues as you grapple with infertility, then seeing someone one-on-one may be the best option for you. Counselors also are able to help couples communicate more effectively, make important decisions, or resolve the issues of loss that are so intertwined with infertility diagnosis and treatment.

Let me begin by exploring the different types of professionals who are there to help you. These terms cover a wide range of professionals:

Psychiatrists, who are MDs, can provide a diagnosis (especially when you are dealing with feelings of depression and anxiety), and they can recommend and write prescriptions for medication. (Always make careful inquiries about the possible effects of any medication on a developing fetus.) Some psychiatrists offer counseling, but it is likely that they will refer you to one of the other professionals in this list.

Psychologists, all of whom have master's degrees and many of whom have PhDs, cannot prescribe medication, but they have been educated in how to assess your strengths and limitations in coping. Their counseling expertise has been gained through coursework, clinical internships, and post-degree supervised clinical experience.

Social workers, who will have at least a master's degree, may also have other credentials attesting to their expertise in clinical counseling. Their counseling expertise, acquired through coursework, an internship, and possibly post-degree supervised clinical experience, is often supplemented by skills in promoting couple communication, addressing issues of loss, advocacy, and connecting clients with appropriate community resources.

Marriage and family therapists, who will have at least a master's degree, may also have other credentials attesting to their experience in clinical counseling. Their counseling expertise in marriage and family issues is acquired through coursework, an internship, and possibly post-degree supervised clinical experience.

You can find a counselor in many ways. Since ideally you want a counselor who has some familiarity with infertility, you might ask any infertile friends if they know of counselors in your area who have been helpful to them. If you prefer to be more anonymous, you can contact the IAAC or RESOLVE (see this book's Resources section) to inquire about finding a local chapter. Other resources may be your local mental health society, your clergy, your ob-gyn, or the social worker at your community hospital.

Once you have found your potential counselor, you will need to ask a few questions:

Can the counselor see me right away, or is there a waiting list?
If you are not feeling a sense of urgency and are willing to wait, at least ask whether you could have an initial interview with the counselor soon so that both of you can assess if you would be compatible. If you don't feel comfortable with the counselor, keep looking until the fit feels right. If the outcome of that meeting is positive, ask when you can set up regular appointments. If the time frame seems too long, ask the counselor whether she or he can recommend another counselor in the community.

What fee does the counselor charge?
Some counselors have a sliding fee scale, so it is appropriate to inquire about the flexibility of the fee. Counselors charge by the session (usually 50 minutes), and many of them will expect that you pay at the end of each session, even if you need to wait to be reimbursed by your insurance carrier.

Will my health insurance cover counseling? Is there a limit to the number of sessions that it will cover?
Before even committing to a counselor, be clear with your insurance carrier about both of these questions. On your first visit to the counselor, tell her or him what, if anything, your insurance

will cover, so the counselor knows what you can afford and you don't spend too much time on finances (time that could be spent talking about your infertility issues).

How frequently will my counseling sessions occur?
Most counselors offer weekly appointments. However, in times of crisis, more frequent appointments can be arranged. If you and the counselor decide that less frequent appointments would serve your needs, you can organize that as well.

How can I reach the counselor between regular appointments?
You may have an urgent issue that cannot wait for your next appointment, or you may simply need to cancel an appointment due to illness, a medical appointment, or some unanticipated event. Most counselors have answering machines that they check regularly — this is so phone calls do not interrupt them when they're with a client. However, the best strategy is to ask the counselor how she or he prefers to be contacted. (This is also a time to inquire about the coverage that your counselor arranges for clients when she or he is out of town.)

What is the counselor's perspective on seeing both me and my partner?
This question is relevant because many counselors will want to meet — at least initially — with your partner and you together. If you and your partner have already decided that you want counseling as a couple, it is important to know whether the counselor is comfortable working with couples.

The Counseling Experience

If you have not seen a counselor before, you are probably wondering what takes place during a session. The exact approach will vary with each counselor, but it is reasonable to expect that in the initial few sessions, the counselor will encourage you to present your perspective on the issues that you're struggling with. She may ask what you have done to cope and what problem-solving strategies you have used so that she can understand how you approach problems, as well as know what has worked and what hasn't. She will probably ask about your support network and the sources of stress in your life.

The counselor may give direct advice, but many counselors are more likely to ask something like "I wonder what would happen if . . . ?" or "Have you ever thought about doing X?" In that way the counselor can gauge from your response whether you would be willing to try a new approach, or whether the people in your life would be responsive to different behavior from you.

Because so much of infertility involves issues of loss, there are likely to be times when you will find yourself in tears as you describe the sadness, anguish, and mourning that you are experiencing. Almost all counselors expect that raw emotions will surface in counseling sessions, and undoubtedly there will be a box of tissues nearby. You need not feel apologetic about showing emotion with a counselor; your capacity to feel and to share those emotions allows the counselor to better understand the depth of your pain. All counseling professionals expect that their clients are encountering difficult times, and they do not expect you to be coping well on your first visit. After all, they know that your reason for seeking help is to share your pain, to learn new coping skills, to make important decisions, and to emerge from the infertility experience a more resilient person or couple.

The experience of counseling will differ for each person. With the several hundred women and men whom I have counseled, I have found that some needed a sympathetic ear and reassurance that I appreciated how stressful infertility had made their lives. Some needed to learn new communication skills that could ease their relationship with their partner and other loved ones. Some needed to weigh the options in undergoing a new medical procedure or to face that, after many tries at the same medical procedure, they needed to move forward in making new decisions. Some needed my encouragement to become more assertive with staff at their infertility clinic (and in several situations, I got my clients' permission to intervene and alert a clinic that staff was behaving rudely or inappropriately with my clients). Some needed to anticipate difficult events and think through how they would handle them, and some needed to be challenged to try new behaviors. But all, at one time or another, needed to hear from me that they were making good decisions, that they were entitled to the emotions they were experiencing, and that they were coping in constructive ways despite the pain of their infertility.

People who have experienced a pregnancy loss, whether an abortion, a fetal reduction, a miscarriage, an ectopic pregnancy, or a stillbirth, will find that counseling can provide an emotional cushion for grieving. Not only will the counselor not expect you to "pull yourself together" or to "accept that it is for the best," as many friends and families may advise, she or he will be patient and accepting of your grief. Many counselors have had considerable experience helping people work through their grief after a loss, and they will understand that you and your partner may have quite different ways of coming to terms with your loss. Since the losses associated with infertility are neither recognized nor ritualized in our society, you may find that the counselor can help you think through how to memorialize your pregnancy loss in a way that has special meaning for you.

Infertility is a condition that encourages you to focus on your body. Whether you are preoccupied with your menstrual cycle, diagnostic tests, medications, test results, side effects, or your ultimate success in becoming pregnant and delivering a healthy baby, the body and its reproductive capacity are central to every person who grapples with infertility. The health professionals with whom you interact will reinforce this. They may inquire about how you're doing, but their expertise is more with your physical health than your emotional health. So it is up to you to recognize that this journey along the pathway of infertility will require emotional resilience. You have sought the best medical care; now you will also need to remind yourself that getting professional help for your emotional health is critical to your capacity to weather the frustrations, disappointments, and anguish of the infertility experience.

Therapeutic Tips

In the preceding chapters of this book I have emphasized the importance of clarifying your emotional needs and taking care of yourself. In this chapter I broaden my emphasis to remind you of people who are well prepared to work *with* you to ensure that you are not overwhelmed by the practical details and the emotional uncertainty of trying to conceive. So perhaps after reading this chapter you're wondering *how* will you know if you need more emotional support than you are getting? Here are some warning signs to watch for:

* Your friends relate to you only in terms of your infertility and the anxiety it causes. If you sense this kind of imbalance in your relationships, a counselor or a support group might be a good place to turn.

- Your partner avoids talking with you about the emotional issues provoked by your diagnosis or treatment. If so, couple therapy would be one way to constructively open up communication channels. If the two of you had decided to lean exclusively on each other for emotional support, this could contribute to your partner feeling overwhelmed or inadequate to meet your needs. In this situation, too, a counselor can help you find different, more balanced ways to cope.

- Your family is either clueless or downright insensitive to your emotional needs. This is a common topic in support group discussions; however, if you think a more personalized approach to your family is what you need, a counselor should be able to look at these family issues and explore with you how you can handle them.

- You find yourself increasingly depressed and unable to take pleasure in events that used to bring you joy or satisfaction. Mood swings are a known side effect of some hormone treatments for infertility. Be sure to discuss with your infertility specialist the occurrence of any serious mood swings; it is possible that a change in medications will reduce the severity of any depression. Depression is an understandable response to the losses and out-of-control feelings associated with infertility treatment. If you can identify a counselor quickly, do so. He or she very likely will have a working relationship with at least one psychiatrist in your community who can evaluate your depression. Ultimately the counselor will continue to work with you regularly, and the psychiatrist may recommend medication to address your depression. Just be sure to discuss with the psychiatrist, your infertility physician, and your pharmacist any possible effects of those medications on a developing fetus. Your counselor is also likely to know of other supportive resources in your community that can help you use mind–body approaches as an antidote to depression: yoga, guided imagery, mindful meditation, relaxation breathing, and acupuncture, to name a few.

- Your group of friends is shrinking because of their dedicated memberships in The Club. An infertility support group can provide both empathy and practical suggestions about how to identify helpful resources, how to bring humor back into your life, and how to keep from being consumed by your struggle to have a baby.

- Your spiritual or religious faith is shaken. This may be a good time to talk with the clergy at your place of worship. If you are not affiliated with a particular place of worship, you may be able to learn from friends about a religious leader who can empathize with issues of loss. If attending several worship services provides you with reassurance that you could approach this religious leader, do so and see whether he or she provides the guidance and spiritual comfort you need.

Eight

Pregnancy Loss:
A Shattered Dream

Losing a pregnancy causes anguish for women and their partners. Infertile women never take for granted the capacity to become pregnant, nor do they assume that a pregnancy will result in a healthy birth. They've experienced too many disappointments and are highly sensitive to the possibility of bodily betrayal.

For those who go the route of home pregnancy tests, the pregnancy may have represented a triumph that they would not need to seek more sophisticated medical diagnosis and treatment. For those who used assisted reproductive technologies (ART), this pregnancy followed many medical procedures, disruptions in schedules, financial sacrifices, and always an effort to be hopeful about the outcome. Regardless of the circumstances of the pregnancy, its loss is an excruciating end to the dreams of a baby, of parenthood, of membership in The Club, and of nurturing the family's next generation.

Types of Fetal Loss

Fetal loss can occur any time in a pregnancy and in many different ways. A loss before the hCG level has climbed is usually referred to as the loss of a *chemical pregnancy* (hCG, or human chorionic gonadotropin, is a hormone that increases early in the pregnancy); a loss that occurs in the first 20 weeks is known as a *miscarriage* or a *spontaneous abortion*; an embryo that begins to develop outside the uterus (often in a fallopian tube) and requires surgical removal to save the life of the mother is an *ectopic pregnancy*; the abortion of one or more fetuses in a multiple pregnancy is known as *multifetal pregnancy reduction*; the death of the fetus between the twentieth week and birth is termed a *stillbirth*. Some women experience multiple losses if they are pregnant with multiples and they lose some or all of the fetuses, or if they have repeat miscarriages or repeat stillbirths.

With infertility as a backdrop to pregnancy loss, it can be especially devastating, as it not only represents the loss of a baby but also reinforces the woman's perception that her body cannot be counted on to carry a pregnancy to a healthy birth.

Infertile couples have been conditioned not to get their hopes up, but once they get a positive pregnancy test, they inevitably hope for a healthy baby. Since many women have nurtured dreams of a baby for months or even years, a pregnancy provides a joyful focus for those fantasies.

And from that focus grows an attachment to the baby, minuscule as it may be. Ultrasounds and the photographs of the baby in utero have allowed you to see your new little miracle. Although you know at a rational level that not all pregnancies lead to a healthy birth, you still believe that after trying so long and so hard, certainly *this* pregnancy deserves to be healthy. Not only is the fantasy of the baby increasingly powerful, so is the fantasy of becoming a parent.

At whatever point the pregnancy ends, the losses are profound. The baby is gone; the role of parent will never be experienced with this child; the hopefulness of grandparents- and aunts- and uncles-to-be evaporates, and you must once again face the world with an ache in your heart. Since there are no rituals to mark a pregnancy loss, you are especially likely to feel isolated in your grief. If you had not yet shared the news of your pregnancy, then there may be few people to support you emotionally.

Grief, Guilt, Regret, and Anger

Grief over a lost pregnancy inevitably comes with many other emotions. There is desperation, fear of getting older, stress over watching the savings account dwindle, worries over how many more mood swings you and your partner can weather, and questions about how much more medical intervention your body can take.

Many women experience feelings of guilt and search relentlessly to find a cause for the loss of the baby. They often blame themselves. When the baby is lost, it is understandable to examine whether something you did contributed to the loss or whether you might have done something to prevent this tragic outcome. Especially for women whose pregnancies were achieved through ART, it is tempting to feel at fault, since the medical aspects of the pregnancy were being watched so carefully. So women who earlier reveled in keeping charts and records now find themselves scrupulously examining their every move, every meal, every lift of a heavy object to identify what they did that could have caused the pregnancy to end. It is common to wonder whether using reproductive technologies might have contributed to the fate of the pregnancy. This question is especially troubling for women whose religions oppose assisted reproductive technologies and who wonder if God is punishing them for not observing their religion's teachings.

Guilt also can extend to past behaviors that you now regret. If you experienced the termination of an earlier, unplanned pregnancy, your current pregnancy loss is likely to seem like retribution. If a sexually transmitted infection left you with scarred tubes or reproductive organs, you may regret lack of attention to sexual health. If you delayed childbearing to meet other life goals, you may feel it's a cruel irony that a child really would be the most precious life goal to achieve. In some cases, either partner may be in a second marriage, at last ready to begin a family; the regret at time spent in an earlier relationship can also fuel guilt when you and your partner encounter infertility and pregnancy loss.

Anger is an emotion that is closely intertwined with grief. After enduring the sadness and frustration of infertility, only to be emotionally assaulted with the loss of a pregnancy, you may feel furious that you are being singled out for such thwarted life dreams. Yet a target for your anger is not close at hand. You may feel angry at the health-care professionals whom you suspect did not do everything possible to ensure a healthy pregnancy. But given the likely dependence on the same medical staff for future conceptions, you probably will not express your anger openly. You may be angry with God for punishing you, but the result may be a spiritual isolation from your religious leader or friends in the congregation. Your anger may even be directed at the baby who died in utero. As one mother said, "Couldn't he just have hung in there for nine months?" Even though the targets of the anger may not seem especially rational, there is no question that women and men who experience a pregnancy loss are entitled to feel angry and cheated of a life hope that so many take for granted. Just remember that it is important not to displace that anger into relationships with loved ones.

Reactions of Family and Friends

So let's talk about the important loved ones in your life — your partner, your parents, siblings, in-laws, and friends, who may have shored you up during the months or years of hoping for this pregnancy. Not only do you have your own grief to bear, but you also must figure out how you are going to relate to your support network, balancing your need for privacy and your need for empathic listeners and shoulders to lean on.

Because there is such a discomfort with grief in North American society, even loved ones may minimize the emotional pain associated with this loss. It is common for friends and relatives to reassure a couple by reminding them that at least now they know they can achieve a pregnancy. Some people, believing that a fetal abnormality contributed to the miscarriage, will suggest that "this was for the best" or "you can always try again." These remarks, in addition to being ill-informed, minimize the loss of the baby and further isolate you from the support you need. When you experience a number of insensitive responses, you begin to question whether you even are entitled to mourn.

Early Loss

A positive pregnancy test is hoped-for, but unexpected. Since this pregnancy has been so hard to conceive, you are likely to cherish every single day, even as you are aware at some level that the first several months of a pregnancy can be precarious.

So you are watchful, tentatively joyful, quietly apprehensive, appreciating each day that the pregnancy continues. But then a day comes when you are no longer pregnant, and your world falls apart. Here are the experiences of women who share the anguish of losing an early pregnancy:

"I was ecstatic when my home pregnancy test turned out positive! But of course I didn't trust it, so I went to Planned Parenthood and had them do a test, and when that one came back positive I just cried for joy. We had been trying for about two years, and we were just on the verge of going to an infertility clinic for a workup. I was relieved that this pregnancy meant we didn't have to go that route. But after a few weeks, when I began to have cramps, my doctor warned me that I might be facing a miscarriage. She suggested bed rest, which I did for two weeks, but the pains kept coming, and late one night I passed a lot of blood. That was it. No drama, no medical emergency, but my life felt so empty. The doctor did a D&C [dilation and curettage] and told me to wait a couple of months before trying again, but I'm so shattered I can't even look that far ahead. Reed keeps saying it is a good sign that I was able to get pregnant, but all I can focus on is how long it took and how I'm not getting any younger. I'm just consumed with the sadness of losing this baby. Trying to get pregnant again won't erase from my mind and my heart that my baby died before it could even have a chance at life. So how am I coping? It's hard to say, but one thing that helps is talking about my sadness, and I'm lucky that I have friends and family who are understanding and willing to listen. I'm trying to figure out whether I have the patience and optimism to try to get pregnant again before we go to an infertility clinic. I guess I'd like to know from some specialists if there is a biological reason that getting pregnant and staying pregnant is so hard for me. Once I have answers to those questions, it will be easier to figure out what next steps to take."

"You know, with all the medical tests and procedures I've undergone, I'd made a big investment in this pregnancy. At some level I guess I felt that since I couldn't do this by myself, perhaps having the best doctors in the city would ensure a healthy pregnancy. And in the beginning, when they told me I was pregnant, I felt that we had made the right choice to sink so much time and money into IVF [in vitro fertilization]. But as the clinic monitored my hCG levels, the nurses were more and more cautious with each communication. Finally, when the levels fell too low, they told me that this pregnancy would not continue. I don't even feel as if I'm entitled to mourn, since they say that I only had a 'chemical pregnancy.' But in my heart, even for just that week, I believed I was going to have a baby. And the sadness I feel is more than a chemical mood swing. So now we have to figure out what's next and whether there is anything the doctors learned from this that will make them more optimistic about another IVF attempt. In the meantime, I'm shedding some quiet tears each day, trying to pamper myself by splurging on funky jewelry and some of my favorite comfort foods. I've also joined a RESOLVE support group, and it really helps to be with these women and couples who also are struggling to move forward with their lives."

"The term *ectopic pregnancy* wasn't anything I had ever heard of. After all these months of trying to get pregnant, both my doctor and I were thrilled when the pregnancy test turned out positive. And, of course, Dan was just ecstatic. He had put up with my worrying and my charts and my calendars for so long. It was a joy to begin to plan for this baby instead of worrying that I couldn't get pregnant. And then out of the blue came this incredible pain like nothing I'd ever experienced before. I didn't really think it had anything to do with the baby — I thought it was appendicitis. When we got to the emergency room and they diagnosed an ectopic pregnancy, I didn't know what they were talking about. They had to move me into surgery so quickly that I didn't learn until later that I had lost both the baby and my right fallopian tube, which was ready to burst when they operated. The doctor and everyone else kept telling me that I'm lucky to be alive, but I keep asking how lucky is it to have lost a baby and a fallopian tube that could help me to have another baby? So now I'm trying to slow down, to take care of myself, and to do lots of reading on infertility. But my friend who has been trying for years to get pregnant warned me against getting consumed by my infertility. So she and I have a pact that we'll meet a couple of times a month for lunch or coffee and we'll share what we've been doing to have fun, to soothe ourselves, and to be thoughtful to other people who have their own troubles. There's no question that a big focus in the coming months will be on trying to get pregnant, but I also need to work at keeping my perspective."

"When I had a miscarriage at four weeks, it was practically a non-event for everyone but Ben and me. Since we already have a six-year-old daughter, no one has ever taken very seriously that I'm grappling with secondary infertility. They know I'm trying to get pregnant, but they also see the joy that Lisa brings into our lives, so they assume that I'm fulfilled as a parent. Of course I am in many ways, but my fantasy family always included two or three kids. And now that Lisa has been asking for a couple of years why I don't have a brother or a sister for her, I also feel like I'm not the only one to want a larger family. In retrospect, I'm glad that Ben and I agreed not to tell Lisa about the pregnancy so early, because I really don't want to have her involved in our preoccupation with having more children. I've decided that I'm going to try to find a therapist who can help Ben and me sort out our feelings about this miscarriage and the shattered dream it represents."

Loss after the First Trimester

Once the first trimester has passed, and with it the greatest likelihood of losing this pregnancy, you are likely to relax more fully and to begin to take pleasure in being pregnant. By now you have felt flutters of life, you may be wearing your first maternity clothes, you are sharing your news with everyone in sight, and you are feeling round and maternal. And then your life is shattered as you lose this pregnancy. Women and their partners who share this experience are devastated, as is evident in the following scenarios:

"I am still so devastated by this miscarriage that I can barely talk about it without breaking down into tears. After all the tests and treatments and after five months of pregnancy, I had really allowed myself to hope that, at long last, I was going to become a mother. I had been wearing maternity clothes for a couple of weeks, so people were asking me about the due date and how I was feeling, and it was just wonderful to be able to share my joy with everyone from best friends to store clerks. To lose this baby is just more than I can bear. Of course I've spent a lot of time wondering whether there was something I did — something I ate, some toxic fumes I was exposed to, some physical exertion, but I can't think of anything. I took the remains of the miscarriage to my doctor, but he was unable to determine anything.

So here I am, with my hopes and dreams in shambles. At first I didn't want to leave the house except to go to work. People at the office were sympathetic, but they have their busy lives and now that a month has passed they've pretty much moved on. But now when I go to the grocery store with all the babies being pushed through the aisles, and to the mall with pregnant women and strollers everywhere, I am reminded of the joy that I have lost. So I've told Jerry that I need him to do more shopping, and I am trying each day to take walks in a nearby park where I can steer clear of the playground. I've begun to find some solace in nature and its beauty, and I'm becoming more comfortable with being alone and accepting that this sadness is now a part of me. In a way I say to myself that this baby would not want to have me carry this sadness forever, so I'm gradually trying to shape my life around things that make me smile: music, flowers, chocolate, and nature. I've talked a lot with Jerry about what I'm doing to try to heal, partly because he needs to figure this out for himself and partly because I don't want him to think that he has to cheer me up. We're even discussing getting a dog — not as a baby substitute, but as something to love and have fun with at home. So, who knows? Even though I still feel incredible emotional pain, I know that we will get through this and hopefully become parents someday."

"One of the worst things about losing our baby at six months has been the number of people who hadn't seen me in awhile and who assumed I had given birth. So what do you do when someone gives you a big smile or a hug and says, 'Congratulations! Is it a boy or a girl?' Of course my eyes would well up with tears and I'd tell them that we lost the baby, and the whole situation was terribly awkward. I would be a wreck for days, wondering how many more times this was going to happen. I almost became a recluse, but my mother insisted that I get myself out of the house each day. She told me to practice in front of a mirror what I would say the next time I ran into someone who assumed the baby had arrived. I had a whole paragraph memorized, and I did feel more in control with words on the tip of my tongue. My mother knows that being in control is important to me. Her help after the miscarriage was so comforting. She cautioned me that people would try to comfort me with words that offered little comfort, and she was right. I had to figure out how to respond to thoughtless or painful remarks, because to ignore them felt so false. So now when people tell me they're sure it was for the best or they wonder if it wouldn't be a good idea to adopt, I'm able to let them know that I'm still feeling a lot of grief over this baby and I'd appreciate their sympathy rather than their suggestions. As I think about how I'm grieving, I guess I'd have to say that I'm trying to talk a bit about the sadness and at the same time not to let it drown me. I can only hope that I am able to get pregnant again, and when that happens I intend to tell my doctor that he should treat the pregnancy as high risk from the beginning. But for today and tomorrow and next week, the best I can do is to stay in touch with my sadness when I feel it and open my heart to new things that will bring me joy."

Loss in a Multiple Pregnancy

Couples who have grappled with infertility and who have sought treatment through ART are often dumbfounded with the news that the woman is carrying multiple fetuses. It seems unreal to move from a place of barrenness to a place in which two, three, or even more embryos have implanted in the woman's uterus. After the initial shock, the couple will discuss with the medical team the risks associated with carrying the pregnancies to term. Those couples who believe that multiple births will provide an instant family, or those whose funds would not have allowed them to continue infertility treatment, may discuss the risks optimistically. Other couples, who feel overwhelmed at the prospect of multiples, will be apprehensive as they weigh with the health team the issues they now face. Once a couple comprehends the potential complications during pregnancy, the possibility of premature delivery, and the higher risk of birth defects in multiples, discussions with the medical team focus on how to maximize the health of both mother and babies.

Loss in multiple gestation can occur as an early miscarriage; as a result of fetal reductions; as a loss later in the pregnancy; or may be detected as an ultrasound reveals a change in the number of gestational sacs. The uniqueness of pregnancy loss with multiples is that there still may be the delivery of at least one baby, which leaves parents with the haunting feeling that their family is not quite complete. Another more tragic possibility is that all the fetuses are lost, leaving the couple grief-stricken and bereft. The feelings of loss mirror in many ways those of previously infertile women carrying single pregnancies, but the loss is compounded by unique factors: the extent of medical monitoring of this high-risk pregnancy; the extent of accommodations that the woman has made to ensure the health of the pregnancy; and the emotional capacity of the couple to mourn the loss of each of the babies.

A unique issue that couples carrying multiples face is whether to reduce the number of fetuses. This choice is devastating. The couple must decide whether to abort one or more fetuses to enhance the health and safety of the remaining fetus or fetuses or to keep them all, but with much greater risk to their health and survival. The backdrop of infertility is a constant reminder to couples of how they cherish each fetus and are unable to view their decision strictly in terms of medical risk. Couples inevitably feel guilty if they decide to reduce the numbers of fetuses in the pregnancy. Since they never can know whether their decision ultimately contributed to the health of the mother and the remaining fetuses, they are faced with nagging doubts at having made an irreversible decision. In the following stories women talk about their experiences of loss while carrying multiples:

"Larry and I were blown away when the doctor told us I was carrying triplets, but we had a lot of confidence in the doctors to monitor the pregnancy and to continue to take good care of me. Imagine our dismay when, at one of our ultrasound appointments, the doctor concluded there was only one heartbeat. As we looked at the monitor we could see three embryos, but two of them were still, while the third clearly had a heartbeat. We barely heard the doctor as she explained that this sometimes happens. All we could feel was that we had lost two of our babies before we even could hold them in our arms. And then, to add to our grief, all our families did was focus on the health of the remaining embryo — altogether ignoring the fact that we were still shedding tears for the babies we had lost."

"The prospect of having twins brought joy into our lives after four years of infertility treatments. I followed the doctors' orders to the letter — I rested, I meditated, I ate carefully. And then at three months I had a miscarriage and lost both of our babies. We're devastated, and I feel so empty with no flutters of life, no dreams to dwell on. I'm overwhelmed by the feeling that this may have been the only time I will ever become pregnant. Everyone tries to comfort us by saying that at least IVF worked, but I can't even begin to contemplate another IVF until I've mourned for these babies."

"When I miscarried one of our twins at 10 weeks, I was overwhelmed with emotions. I was grief-stricken at losing one baby, and I was also terrified that I might lose the remaining twin. So at the very time that I knew I should focus on being calm for the sake of my ongoing pregnancy, I was crying myself to sleep each night and having a lot of trouble focusing during the day. Dave tried to be comforting, but he was also scared that dwelling too much on our loss would endanger my ability to bond with our baby who was still growing inside me. Finally we decided to see a therapist, since we just couldn't get past the sadness of one loss and the worry that it might happen again. The therapist helped us to focus on our grief for a little time together each day, which was very soothing for both of us. She also helped us to decide what questions we needed to ask our doctors about the health of our remaining baby. Once we learned more clearly from the doctor the answers to our questions, we used that approach on each prenatal visit to get a sense of some control. Even though we were always aware that the pregnancy was high risk, being able to talk about it with our therapist gave us the ongoing sense we were doing all we could do. Heaven forbid that anything more should happen, but if it does, at least I'll be comforted knowing that we did everything possible to take care of ourselves and this baby."

"When the IVF clinic called to say I was pregnant, Jerry and I were ecstatic. We had spent our savings on earlier IVFs and we couldn't believe that I was pregnant on what would be our last try. But soon we learned that all five embryos had implanted, and both of us were on the verge of heart attacks! There was no way we could possibly raise five children born at the same time. The doctors, who were looking at my pregnancy more from a medical perspective, suggested that we reduce some of the fetuses to give the remaining ones a better chance to develop to full term. At first this made sense but, pro-choice as I am, it just felt wrong to make such a matter-of-fact decision about 'reducing' the number of babies that I would have. Since I am small boned to begin with, the doctors said that even if I carried twins there was a likelihood of premature labor. So Jerry and I told the doctors that we wanted them to select the embryo that looked the strongest and to abort the others. Once the procedure was over, we both felt so sad. I keep wondering if we were being selfish about wanting to maximize our chances of having at least one healthy baby. I keep thinking that after our child is born, I'll probably see four phantom siblings playing on the swing set in our backyard."

"Never in my life have I been so confused as I was when our daughter was born prematurely and her twin brother was stillborn. Within minutes of one nurse asking us if we wanted to hold our son before they took his body to the morgue, another nurse appeared to ask if I was ready to visit my daughter in the nursery. I would have known how to react to the events separately, but having them occur together was just too much. We ultimately sent two announcements to our friends — the first being the birth of our daughter and the second being the birth and death of our son. After we brought our daughter home from the hospital everyone focused on her health and cuteness, and Don and I seemed to be the only ones who remembered that we had lost our beloved son. Within a couple of weeks we had a small service in Matt's memory, and preparing for that helped us begin to heal. But I just know that when we celebrate Sarah's birthdays, it will be a bittersweet time for Don and me."

Stillbirth

Stillbirth is one of the most devastating experiences that an infertile couple can endure. Whether the baby dies before labor begins, during labor, or during delivery, most couples are completely unprepared for such a tragic outcome to this precious pregnancy. Even though the backdrop of infertility leaves most women very cautious about their capacity to conceive and to carry a healthy pregnancy to term, many women let out a figurative sigh of relief after the first trimester, when most miscarriages occur. Unless she has experienced complications in the pregnancy, or unless she has experienced an earlier pregnancy loss, most women assume that each month brings a heightened likelihood of a healthy baby. Sometimes it is the woman who identifies the warning signs: too many hours with no fetal movement, spotting, cramping, or the onset of premature labor. In other situations, a prenatal visit is the time at which the doctor is unable to detect a fetal heartbeat and must tell the woman that her baby has died. This news precipitates shock and grief as the couple tries to reconcile their previous hopes and dreams with the reality that they will never be able to welcome this baby into the world with joy. Instead they must prepare for the eventual labor and delivery of their dead child.

At this time most women and their partners are mired in confusion and anguish. When they learn that the baby cannot be delivered until labor begins spontaneously or until it can be induced, they face the specter of returning home still visibly pregnant but carrying a load of grief that seems insurmountable. The couple must consider how to tell family members, how to handle questions about the pregnancy from people the woman encounters in the days before the onset of labor, and how to think about putting this baby to rest after it is delivered. Many women want to seclude themselves from the empathic smiles that a pregnant belly elicits, from the presence of pregnant women and infants that once again are unbearable, and from the expectation she senses that she should greet the world with a joyful smile. Many women experience profound ambivalence about carrying a dead baby. On the one hand, both parents can be prepared for the grief they will experience when labor begins. On the other hand, the pain of knowing that one's baby did not survive causes many women to wish that the delivery could be over so they can stop dreading it. The following accounts show how some women have experienced and coped with the tragedy of a stillbirth:

"Last month I called the doctor's office to say that I hadn't felt the baby move for at least eight hours. Since I was seven months along and this was a very active baby, I was worried. The nurse asked me to come right in and there was something in her voice that made me call Jim and tell him to meet me at the doctor's office. We arrived at just the same time, and the nurse showed us right in to an examining room. She said that the doctor would be right in, but that she would get me prepped for the fetal monitor. As she moved the device across my belly, listening for the heartbeat, she couldn't find one. By then Jim and I were frantic, and we demanded that the doctor be brought in right away. The nurse disappeared and by the time the doctor arrived I was in tears. He tried to find a heartbeat and couldn't. The rest of the afternoon is a blur. I remember being told that our baby had died and being offered the choice of whether to have labor induced or to wait until it began spontaneously. We were in complete disbelief, but we both knew we needed time to be alone and to call our families. The next few days were pure agony. I cannot describe what it was like to carry a baby that I had grown to love, that was a real part of our lives, and to know it was dead and there was nothing I could do to bring it back. When the labor began, my father drove Jim and me to the hospital, while my mother followed in their car. It was such a comfort to have my parents there, both for the birth of our dead baby and for all they did to try to ease our pain. My parents asked if we wanted to have a minister visit in the hospital, if we wanted to have a service to memorialize the baby, and even if we wanted to give him a name. But more helpful than anything, they ran the house and the kitchen while Jim and I lay in our hammock in the backyard trying to figure out where our lives would go from here. As I look back over the past four weeks, I still feel the raw pain. Once I had taken as much sick leave from work as I could afford, I tried to get back into a routine that wasn't too hectic. Mom had left a lot of cooked dinners in the freezer, and she and Dad had left us a generous check with instructions to get out of town for some weekend trips. And with them calling us each day, we were assured that if we really fell apart they would be there in a minute. To my surprise, I did not fall apart, but I still feel an enduring sadness that I don't think will ever leave. Jim and I have decided to plant a memorial garden in our son's memory in the backyard, and as we draw up the designs, I feel calm. Our due date will be coming up soon, and I have already told Jim we must use that date to begin planting. I hope the garden will become a quiet place for both of us to sit and enjoy the beauty that it brings."

"When the contractions began, I had no idea what was happening. After trying so long to become pregnant, I was an expert on infertility, but I was still reading the small library that I'd acquired on pregnancy. None of the books on the last trimester of pregnancy prepared me for labor to begin early in the seventh month. So when the pains began I thought I might be constipated. I was on the telephone with my sister when one of the contractions hit, and she was immediately suspicious. She insisted that I call my obstetrician, which I did, and I was told to come right to the office. When I got there, the doctor said that I was definitely experiencing contractions. He had been my doctor through all our infertility efforts, so he knew how precious this baby was to us. He told me that he was going to hospitalize me and put me on medication that would hopefully eliminate the contractions and allow me to carry the pregnancy until it was closer to my delivery date. But after three days in the hospital with weak contractions, suddenly they became stronger and my water broke. I could tell from the look on the doctor's face that this was the end, and he gently told me that our baby could not survive. Of course I knew nothing about labor and delivery so, although the nurses tried to help me breathe through the contractions, I had a very hard time. I know it was worse because I was overwhelmed with grief. After the delivery, the doctor let Bob and me hold the baby until we were ready to say goodbye, and then to my shock I was moved to a room on the maternity wing. The nurses thought they were doing us a favor by putting me in a single room, but it took hours before we were able to get my doctor to intervene and have me placed on another floor, away from crying babies, nursing mothers, and proud grandparents. The hospital stay was just the beginning of letting go of our dreams. When I got home I found the nursery as yet another reminder of the emptiness in my life. Bob and I agreed that we needed to put the baby things away ('for another time,' we consoled ourselves), so over the next week we gently tucked away clothes, diapers, and stuffed toys and took apart the cradle and changing table. Dismantling the nursery was heartbreaking, but at some level it was also a concrete acknowledgment that our baby had died. I cried more packing up the nursery than I did at the hospital, where my main emotions were anger and frustration about the maternity ward."

"I had been at the obstetrician's office the day before my labor began, and everything seemed fine. Naturally, with our history of infertility, I was feeling anxious as we approached the due date. I was worried about how I'd handle the labor and delivery and whether I'd be a good parent, but those worries were mild compared to what lay ahead. As soon as my water broke, the doctor told us to drive to the hospital. We were both excited and tense. We called our parents on the cellphone on our way to the hospital and told them to wait for our call about their new grandchild. When we got to the hospital and into the labor room, they hooked me up to a fetal monitor. My contractions were getting closer and closer together, so Tom and I were concentrating on my breathing, and we didn't notice the nurses' concern as they summoned the doctor. When he arrived and looked at the readings from the monitor, he said the baby was in serious distress and would need to be delivered by Cesarean section. We were shocked that something seemed to be so seriously wrong, but we told him to do whatever he could to save the baby. The anesthesiologist put me under, and the next thing I remember is seeing Tom's tearful face. I knew then that we had lost our precious baby. When the doctor came in, he explained that the umbilical cord had been wrapped around the baby's neck and strangled her. So in one sentence I learned that our baby had been a little girl and that she had died. I just couldn't stop crying, so they gave me a sedative, and the next time I woke up, my parents were there and Tom's were on the way. Once I was fully conscious, the nurse explained that we could have some time alone with our daughter's body, as a way to say goodbye to her. I reminded the nurse that I hadn't even seen my baby yet, so how could I be expected to say goodbye? I felt so inadequate. I would have known what to do if she had been handed to me alive and healthy after she was born. But there's no way to know how to do what we eventually did — hold our dead baby and explain to her that we would have done anything to save her. We told her how much our love for her had grown during her time inside me and that we would always remember her. But deep inside I was feeling like a powerless mother, not strong enough to save my own child from dying. First I couldn't get pregnant and when I finally did, I delivered a dead baby. Intellectually I know I had no control over the cord wrapping around her neck, but emotionally I know that as a mother I failed to protect my baby. I have a hard time believing that I will ever deserve to be a mother."

It is hard to believe that, at the very time you are grieving the loss of your baby to stillbirth, you must make decisions. You may be asked if you want some mementos of your baby, such as a lock of hair, a photograph, the hospital wristband, or the blanket in which the baby was wrapped. You may consider whether to name the baby, whether to request an autopsy, whether to have a religious service, and how to notify family and friends of the baby's birth and death. The next stories cover some of these difficult decisions:

"The hospital social worker visited with us the day after our son was stillborn. She was very sensitive, and she told us that she wanted to offer herself in whatever way she could be helpful. She mentioned the kinds of decisions that we probably had begun to consider and asked if we would like to talk about them. We decided to ask for her help in learning about burial and cremation options and how to write the obituary, which led into whether or not we would give our baby a name. We hadn't made a final decision when I went into labor. Since it was only my eighth month I thought we had plenty of time. But we had discussed some possible names earlier in the pregnancy, and we finally decided to name our baby Paul, after my grandfather. It somehow became easier to talk about Paul once we had named him. And, in a way, having a name gave him membership in our family, even though he died before we could give him all the love we'd been saving for him."

"When the hospital minister visited us shortly after Melissa was stillborn, we were still in shock. Our families were coming in from out of town, but we were very much alone. We asked the hospital minister to notify the minister of our local church, and she came immediately. She was very comforting, and she helped us to begin thinking about whether we wanted to have a service to honor Melissa's memory. The three of us, with me in a wheelchair, went to the hospital chapel where our minister led us in prayer, and she did that again when our parents arrived. We decided to have a memorial service in the community church, and the minister offered to plan the service and to ask for our input. She was very sensitive to our needs, and she also encouraged members of the congregation to reach out to us, so we felt embraced and cared for spiritually. It was reassuring for our parents to see how members of the congregation supported us with cooked meals, fresh flowers, and offers to run errands. Although we feel empty in our hearts, our minister was able to cushion our pain. She even made an audiotape of the service, so we have that to add to our box of our memories of Melissa."

"While we were in the hospital following Julie's stillbirth, we decided that we just didn't have the strength for a service. We were barely managing around family members who understood our tears and anger, and we weren't ready to be on good behavior in public. Since the stillbirth occurred after seven months and we weren't going to have a service, my mother reminded us that we probably needed to find a way to notify extended family and friends. We decided to have Stan's and my parents call family members, and then Stan and I composed a very brief announcement that we sent to our friends. It said, 'We are so sad to tell you of the stillbirth of our beloved daughter, Julie Marie, on June 1 at Memorial Hospital in Boise, Idaho.'"

Your Partner's Experience of Pregnancy Loss

Although loved ones and acquaintances realize that this loss affects both you and your partner, there is often an assumption that you need more comfort because your body carried the pregnancy. In fact, your partner's initial emotions may have been lost in the medical events that focused primarily on you. In the midst of hospital procedures, your partner may have felt the need to be strong for your sake, and even hospital personnel may have treated your partner as your supporter, rather than acknowledging the grief that both of you shared. If this pattern started in the hospital, then your partner may have assumed the role of the strong supporter and discounted the emotional toll the loss was taking on him or her. Once you are home this role is often reinforced by people asking him or her how *you* are doing, with the tacit assumption that your partner's pain is less than yours.

So in the midst of your own sadness, you will want to acknowledge to others that your partner is grieving this loss too, and ask them to offer verbal and practical support to *both* of you. Although you will, of course, welcome the support that your partner is providing, you will need to look for ways that you, too, can offer support. This may be as simple as initiating some time to hold and comfort one another. It could include asking directly about how your partner's emotions are affecting work, concentration, and relationships. As both of you discuss whether or how to memorialize the baby, it will be important for your partner to take an active part in these decisions. Even if the external world sees your partner primarily in a support-ive role, you both can strengthen your relationship by making a conscious effort to express not only your grief but also the ways you can move forward in the aftermath of this loss.

Therapeutic Tips

The sadness of a pregnancy loss is not measured by the num-ber of months of the pregnancy, but rather by the emotional attachment of the parents-to-be. With a history of difficulty in conceiving, you and your partner have carried a unique hope-fulness. You have known this to be a precious pregnancy, and you probably have felt apprehensions with every twinge and abdominal pain. If you passed your first trimester, you may have even breathed a figurative sigh of relief, looking forward to wearing maternity clothes, to letting others know of this much-wanted pregnancy, and carefully celebrating your new status as "almost parents."

The loss of your baby jolts everyone. You and your partner have needed to decide what loved ones to call immediately, how to make some sense of the meaning of this loss, how to advocate for yourselves in the hospital, how to cope with the enormity of your grief, and how to reach out to each other.

Once home from the hospital, you may find that others want to spare you the grief to which you are entitled. Perhaps well-meaning loved ones have dismantled the baby's nursery; perhaps friends and coworkers tell you you're looking well and they hope life is getting back to normal; perhaps you are encountering acquaintances who haven't heard of your loss and who ask you expectantly whether the baby is a boy or a girl. No matter what the reaction, it is likely that wherever you turn most people lack the words or the empathy to recognize that this loss has changed your lives forever and healing will be gradual.

When you get home, with your pain still fresh, there are some steps you can take to be constructive about your emotional healing:

- If concerned friends and family are treating your partner as a supportive bystander, encourage them to express their sympathies directly and to ask how they can be helpful to *both* of you at this difficult time.

- Remember that there is no one "right" way to grieve, so both you and your partner should be respectful of your differences as you try to make peace with this sadness. Just because it is a shared sadness does not mean that you will grieve the same way, agree on how to move forward emotionally, or even be able to understand where each other is coming from. The important message here is to be open with each other about your own feelings and to be respectful of your partner's different pace, different perspective, or different needs for comfort.

- Be as clear as you can with others (including your partner!) about how they can offer emotional comfort and concrete support. Maybe you simply need to repeat your experience many times to understanding loved ones; maybe you need to have others run errands for a few months in the public places where you know you will encounter pregnant moms and infants; maybe you need help with bills and insurance forms; maybe you need someone to accompany you on your errands so you won't feel so alone; or maybe you need someone to suggest books, Web sites, spiritual sources of strength, or other resources to comfort you. Gather your loved ones around you physically, by e-mail, on social networking Web sites, or by telephone, and let them know how much their love means and how they can support you as you try to heal.

- Anticipate that there will be certain dates and events that may trigger grief. The most powerful one is likely to be your due date. Other days that have the potential to catapult your emotions into a sad place include family gatherings, such as christenings and holidays (see Chapter 6), as well as announcements of pregnancies and births. And then there are the events you never could have anticipated, for example, the "welcome baby" advertisements and small gift samples that arrive in the mail from businesses marketing to expectant moms. Or you could find yourself emotionally unglued with a call from a local diaper service, asking whether you will enroll with them. These events are unanticipated reminders of the different course your life has taken since the time of your pregnancy loss. Give yourself time to breathe deeply, take your emotional pulse, pause to honor the memory of your baby, and take special care of yourself as you regain your emotional equilibrium.

- Find ways to memorialize your baby. You have probably saved items that remind you of him or her. Perhaps you have tucked away an ultrasound, letters from loved ones wishing you well in your pregnancy, a small stuffed animal, or a hand-crocheted blanket. Then there may be more careful plans to memorialize your baby. If you have buried your baby, you may choose a small headstone for the grave. If you did not have a service when your baby died, you may want to plan one. In a society that has no rituals for the often invisible loss of a pregnancy, a remembrance service can comfort you and your partner and loved ones who gather to validate your feelings of attachment to your child. You might want to have a piece of jewelry made as a special keepsake, using your baby's birthstone. If your home has a yard, planting a special flower bed or a tree is another way to create a memorial, but keep in mind that you may not live in your current home forever, so if it would be too painful to leave a garden created with so much love, this plan might not offer long-term comfort.

- Consider doing something positive for your community. You can honor your baby's memory through donations such as books for the public library, baby furniture for a day-care center, or a scholarship for a preschooler to attend a nursery school. A donation to an organization that helps parents cope with the grief of a pregnancy loss may seem especially fitting.

- Create a scrapbook of poems that are meaningful. It may also be comforting to keep a diary of the weeks and months after the pregnancy loss, both as a therapeutic outlet for feelings and as a measure of how far along you have come in resolving your sadness as you move forward.

- Try working with a religious leader or therapist (see Chapter 7) who is comfortable helping people who have experienced loss. Mourning takes time, and as you explore this unfamiliar pathway you may find this helps. Names of therapists can come from the social worker at your local hospital or infertility clinic, from your community mental health clinic or family service agency, or from friends who have had positive experiences with a particular individual. Some hospitals offer support groups for parents who have experienced a pregnancy loss or an infant death. Remember that many therapists will accept insurance or will have sliding fee scales, so don't let financial constraints hold you back from seeking emotional support.

- Know that eventually, since you and your partner will find that your emotional needs evolve and change over time, your conversations will turn to whether or when to try again to conceive. In addition to involving your therapist, you will also want to involve your infertility physician to ask him or her to guide you through the medical options, costs, and other considerations in your decision of whether to pursue treatment.

Nine

Achieving Pregnancy:
An Emotional Roller Coaster

Waiting to learn the outcome of yet another pregnancy test is all too routine for most infertile couples. Whether the test is at home or in a doctor's office, the wait for results evokes anxiety, dread that it will be bad news, memories of earlier negative tests, and the hope beyond hope that this test will be positive. Most infertile women believe that they will receive the news of a pregnancy with joyful relief and be ready to anticipate the remaining months of this much-awaited pregnancy. However, even with the initial joy and relief of a positive pregnancy test (or two!), many women find that the specter of their infertility haunts them in unanticipated ways.

Why Your Pregnancy Feels
Different from Others'

Delightful as it is to be finally in The Club with the legions of pregnant and parenting women who take pregnancy and a healthy delivery for granted, you may sense that your pregnancy — after months or years of infertility — is vastly different from the more easily achieved pregnancies of other women.

First are the emotional hurdles Club members never confronted. They never doubted that they could become pregnant. They never worried that perhaps the birth control they used (or an earlier abortion) might have contributed to their difficulty in getting pregnant. They never obsessed that perhaps they just weren't "meant" to be parents. They never felt guilty that postponing plans for a family to further their educations or careers had placed them at risk of never becoming parents.

Second are the relationship risks and rifts they never negotiated. They never had to bite their tongues at well-meaning but hurtful remarks. They, unlike you, never had to make up endless excuses why they "just couldn't make" a baby shower, a visit to a new mother, or a holiday event. They never needed to stifle jealousy at a sibling's ease at becoming pregnant. They never needed to experience the awkwardness of a pregnant friend who asked, "So what will this mean for our friendship?" They never needed to ask loved ones for a loan for "just one more" medical procedure. They never needed to wonder whether their coworkers resented them because of so many absences for medical procedures. And they never had to tread carefully around health-care professionals who held the key to the elusive dream of becoming pregnant.

Third is that they never endured the unpredictable events of the infertility experience: negative test results, bad side effects of medication, and programmed sex. And it is actually the unpredictable aspects of infertility that are so unbearable. These negative events socialize you to expect bad news, and much of your energy goes into protecting yourself from the sadness that has become such an integral part of your life. Once you understand that you have very little control over your efforts to become pregnant, you are struck by a unique sense of disbelief when you learn that you are, in fact, pregnant! So what does it mean now that you've received the news you've waited so long to hear?

The Many Reactions to Pregnancy

Your unique history of infertility will affect your response to the news of a positive pregnancy test. If your history includes pregnancy losses, you may be wary of becoming joyful too soon for fear that you may lose this pregnancy. If you have had many months of treatment during which you have been very vigilant about your body's responses to drugs, procedures, injections, and the like, you may continue this vigilance as you remain alert to every physical sign of discomfort. In a more positive vein, this much awaited news of your pregnancy may cause you to embrace your new identity and revel in renewing relationships with members of The Club from whom you had distanced yourself.

"On the one hand, I was just terrified. Since I didn't believe that I had anything to do with my success in becoming pregnant, I was at a loss to believe that I could have any effect on keeping this a healthy pregnancy. Every little thing worried me — morning sickness, exhaustion, breast tenderness, even feeling the baby when it first began to move around. In some ways I think I just transferred all the worries of infertility over to my pregnancy. I was in a worrying frame of mind that wasn't going to stop until I had a healthy baby in my arms."

"This is not my first pregnancy. I've had two miscarriages, and so I know I'm going to be fearful until I pass the tenth week, which is when I lost my other two. I don't dare let myself feel the joy I want to feel. I don't dare let myself become attached to this baby. I don't dare begin to think of myself as a mother. Everything emotional feels as if it's on hold until I can be sure that this pregnancy will be a healthy one."

"Both Sean and I are so thrilled — this positive pregnancy test has brought our relationship back to where it was before we began trying to get pregnant. Since his sperm count was so low, we just never knew whether it would be possible for me to conceive with his sperm. Now the prospect of having a baby related to both of us is a dream come true!"

"I wanted to shout the news of my pregnancy from the rooftops! But since I'm single and I've shared my quest for motherhood only with family and close friends, I didn't tell many people about my excitement. But when morning sickness made it necessary to let my coworkers know what was going on, I felt very uneasy — as if I wasn't entitled to my joy and anticipation of being a mother. Happily, once I let everyone know how hard I had been trying to become pregnant, there was a lot of support — mostly from my female coworkers. The guys in the office just seemed confused, but those who have kids seemed more comfortable congratulating me than those who don't."

"The moment I learned I was pregnant, I was determined to savor every minute. I wore maternity clothes long before I needed to, I furnished the nursery with an efficiency that surprised even me, I began going to La Leche League meetings right away so that I would have plenty of time to learn all I could to make nursing a successful experience. And I even began a diary so that, no matter what happened, I couldn't be robbed of remembering the joys of this pregnancy."

Prenatal Testing

In spite of the initial joy of having a positive pregnancy test, you'll find yourself needing to make difficult medical decisions. After finding an obstetrician or a midwife, one of the next decisions is whether to have prenatal testing. Needless to say, after all the infertility tests you have endured, this decision is one that reminds you that pregnancy does not necessarily result in a healthy baby. And with many previously infertile women not conceiving until after age 35, when they are at greater risk of carrying a fetus with chromosomal abnormalities, the availability of prenatal testing is likely to be presented as an option during the first trimester.

For couples undergoing in vitro fertilization (IVF), there is a procedure that can test embryos in the petri dish for chromosomal abnormalities. And for others, about a dozen fetal tests are now available to diagnose birth defects and disease. However, a dilemma arises when technology provides enough information to raise concerns, without providing enough information to make a conclusive diagnosis about the health of the fetus.

The possibility of testing in the first trimester means that couples choosing to terminate the pregnancy can do so early enough that it is less public. But for infertile couples, the issue is to decide what diagnosis would warrant ending a much-wanted pregnancy. And if the diagnosis is problematic, it is unlikely that your discussions will carry much further than the office of your doctor or genetic counselor. After all, you probably don't know anyone who has confronted this decision. And since it is such an emotionally charged decision — ethically, religiously, and personally — it is difficult to discuss with anyone other than your closest loved ones.

One resource for couples who decide to terminate a much-wanted pregnancy is A Heartbreaking Choice, an Internet support group for people who have terminated pregnancies because of the fetus's health.

The bottom line for most couples is how having a child with a particular defect will impact you, your partner, and your family. A closely related consideration is the potential quality of life for the child. The following accounts tell of how some women have struggled with the issues around prenatal testing:

"One of our greatest concerns about prenatal testing was that it might increase the chances of a miscarriage. After all these years of trying to conceive, it would break our hearts if we had a procedure that caused a miscarriage. So we weighed the odds, discussed what it would mean for us to have a baby with birth defects rather than never to become birth parents, and we decided to skip the prenatal testing."

"I had a routine ultrasound late in my first trimester that looked suspicious to my obstetrician. So he sent the ultrasound films to an out-of-town specialist who confirmed that our baby would be born without part of an arm and with stunted legs. There was a possibility of other birth defects as well, but those couldn't be confirmed. I went from the initial ecstasy of being pregnant to shocked depression. Even though we might have been able to handle the physical disabilities, I knew that I could not devote my life to raising a child who might also be mentally challenged. Deciding to terminate the pregnancy was excruciating, and since we presented it to everyone as a miscarriage, I carry that burden with me to this day."

"The toughest thing for me, at age 36, was to imagine what I would do if the prenatal test came back with problems. It turned out that the fetus was diagnosed with Down syndrome. Jeff and I agonized, and ultimately his experience with a cousin having Down syndrome tipped the scales. This cousin, at age 21, still does not speak, is barely toilet trained, and as her parents grow older, they worry about what arrangements they can afford to make for her when they're no longer able to care for her. If that is how our child would develop, I don't think our marriage could survive. We just couldn't take the chance, and we decided to have an abortion and to call it a miscarriage."

"In retrospect, I'm glad that I decided not to broadcast news of our pregnancy until after the fetus was tested for Tay-Sachs, since my husband and I are both carriers and know that the risks for a fetus are high. Neither of us could have dealt with having a baby who would suffer and die in the first couple of years — I mean, who would wish that on a helpless child? So when the diagnosis came back with the results we had dreaded, I had an abortion. We had an informal service at our home in memory of our unborn baby and we grieved for our little angel with our family. Now we're trying to decide whether to try for another pregnancy, which could have the same result, or to pursue adoption."

"Tom and I hadn't known that we were both carriers for cystic fibrosis until after I became pregnant. To have this worry after our years of infertility was just too much! I had an amniocentesis so that the fetus would be tested, and we were just destroyed to learn that our baby would have cystic fibrosis, with progressive lung failure and an average life expectancy of 35 years. The thought of knowingly bringing a baby into this world with serious, and ultimately fatal, health problems was just too much.

We decided to end the pregnancy. We only told close friends and relatives whom we could trust to be supportive, and their love carried us through."

Emotions in the First Trimester

In most pregnancies, previously infertile women find that their emotions are closely timed to the progress of their pregnancy by trimesters. For example, in the first trimester, you may feel joy, but often it is tempered with concern that this is no guarantee of a problem-free pregnancy, a routine delivery, or a healthy baby.

Shifting from your role as an infertile person to someone who actually might become a parent feels like a huge leap of faith. Some women take this leap wholeheartedly, believing that to embrace the pregnancy is to confirm their new status for all to observe. Others are more cautious, especially if they have a long history of reproductive disappointments or pregnancy losses. As the greatest risk of pregnancy loss is during the first trimester, many couples are reluctant to share the news, to become attached to the fetus, or to feel joyful, for fear that such emotions might tempt fate. The physical symptoms in the first trimester can also be disconcerting as morning sickness, nausea, and exhaustion replace the side effects of infertility hormone treatments.

The voices of previously infertile women during their first trimesters clearly articulate both their joy and their apprehension as they anticipate the future of this hoped-for pregnancy:

"I couldn't decide when to share our wonderful news. Fred was all for trumpeting it to the world, but I needed to have some time to think about it more carefully. We had so many friends and family who had been there for us during our infertility. If I told them now and, God forbid, had a miscarriage, I don't think I could bear their disappointment on top of my own grief. A little voice kept telling me to wait until after the first trimester before sharing the news."

"My parents, who love me, were clear for years that they hoped I would end my lesbian relationship and find a husband. But as soon as I became pregnant they indicated in a variety of ways their acceptance of Sherry's and my commitment to each other. I'm pretty sure it is the prospect of being grandparents for the first time that is making them so involved in our lives. Even Sherry is saying that she feels as if my parents have genuinely accepted her."

"Once I left the infertility clinic and was placed under the care of my local ob-gyn, I actually felt even more fragile. At least the professionals in the infertility clinic have a real understanding of how precious this pregnancy is to me. They saw me through the rough times of negative pregnancy tests, mood swings, hormone shots, and even a lapse of insurance coverage. I feel as if everyone in this local office takes this pregnancy for granted and has no understanding of how special it is to me."

"I suddenly realized that this may be my only pregnancy. At a time when I should be filled with joy, I'm finding myself feeling desperate to do everything I can to ensure the health of this pregnancy. I walk gingerly up and down stairs, I eat fruits and vegetables that are organic, I only watch movies with happy endings . . . you get the point. My friends think I'm overdoing it, but after having been able to exert so little control during my infertility treatments, somehow I have the feeling that there are some specific things I can do to make this a healthy pregnancy."

"Since I'm going through this pregnancy as a single person, the moment I became pregnant I began making a special effort to involve my friends and relatives more closely in my life. Not all of them understand why I would want to raise a child as a single mother, but most of them want to be supportive now that I've shared the news of my pregnancy. Interestingly, it seems as if it's up to me to ask for the kind of support I need, which is a bit strange since I've always cherished my independence. But I'm realizing that I want more people in my life as I worry about whether this pregnancy will be healthy, and as I anticipate ways that I'll need support after the baby is born."

"Once Stan and I absorbed this wonderful news, we began to recapture some of the joy in our marriage that had been so badly eroded by the stresses of infertility. And, wouldn't you just know it, after months of programmed sex, where it felt as if our infertility doctor was in bed with us, we had a completely different issue. My obstetrician advised against intercourse during the first trimester! So now that we actually feel in the mood, the doctor tells us we can't make love."

"This pregnancy is different from what I had expected. I'm constantly nauseous, and keeping food down is a real struggle. That makes it hard to function at work, and I'm worried that the nausea is a signal that the pregnancy isn't going well. My doctor tells me that many women have these symptoms early in a pregnancy, but it makes it hard to be excited and confident when I'm feeling so rotten physically."

"Every time I experience a typical symptom of pregnancy, like morning sickness or fatigue, I just smile to myself. It is a reminder to me that I'm *finally* pregnant. There's no way I'll complain about feeling queasy or tired — I've waited so long to be at this place that I'll happily take the bad with the good."

"I'm having such fun being pregnant! I'm reading every book I can find, I'm thinking of what to name the baby, I'm beginning to put together things for the nursery . . . but my one sadness is that Jerry isn't as involved as I expected he would be. He tells me that after our years of infertility he still has trouble believing that we will have a healthy baby. So he is staying emotionally removed so that he can be strong to comfort me if something goes wrong."

Emotions in the Second Trimester

For most women, the second trimester brings a welcome respite from fatigue and nausea. In addition to facing less likelihood of a miscarriage, you also have the joyful experience of feeling the fetus move inside you, hearing its heartbeat, and watching your shape blossom. Conversations about parenthood now take on a more realistic tone: finances, day care, work hours, division of responsibilities, and space issues at home. Parents-to-be who have had little experience with infants may even feel some apprehension about parenting skills.

It is normal for any couple to feel ambivalent as they anticipate their new roles and acknowledge some reservations about the changes that a baby will bring. However, given the efforts they have pursued to become pregnant, many couples will avoid acknowledging any ambivalence, not feeling entitled to anything but joyful emotions after the stress of infertility. The stoicism that had characterized your infertility may discourage you from exploring negative emotions with your partner; consequently, you may shy away from discussing the typical adjustments that most prospective parents face. Instead, you focus on positive thoughts about preparations for the baby's delivery and homecoming.

In addition to anticipating changes on the home front, your pregnancy also may have changed your relationships with friends. The first and second trimesters are times that you may need to renegotiate your relationships with infertile friends, as well as resume any ties with fertile friends that may have been on hold during your infertility. During the second trimester, the ghosts of infertility are less visible. As the following stories show, most women find themselves eager to anticipate the positive changes that will come once they hold a baby in their arms, while others remain nervous about the future of the pregnancy:

"When the baby first fluttered in my uterus, it was the most emotional experience I'd ever had! Better even than the news about the pregnancy test, since the baby's movement makes it real and makes me feel as though there really *is* a baby in there! And now that Chuck can feel it moving too, we are having such a wonderful time anticipating being parents."

"Finally I am showing, and I love it! Now the whole world knows that I'm pregnant, and I'm relishing the questions, the happy wishes, and the attention. And lots of my friends who have children are now much more comfortable being with me than when I was infertile and they were feeling awkward or guilty. Now they are offering me hand-me-downs for the baby's early months and all sorts of pregnancy advice."

"Now that I'm beginning to wear maternity clothes, I'm also getting questions — some from friends who know I will be raising this baby as a single parent, and others from people who are just trying to make conversation. But I certainly feel a little awkward when they ask things like 'And does your husband want a boy?' or 'Be sure to get your husband to do his share of the housework now, so it's not a shock when he needs to pitch in after the baby is born.' But so far I find that a vague smile is all that anyone seems to expect."

"Wearing maternity clothes has brought out some interesting reactions in people who know that I'm in a lesbian relationship. Some are clearly confused and avoid the subject of my pregnancy altogether. Others are curious and open up the subject by congratulating me on my pregnancy and asking about the due date, while clearly hoping I'll offer more information about how I'm going to parent this baby. And then, happily, there are friends who have known all along how carefully we've been trying to conceive and who celebrate this healthy pregnancy with great joy and anticipation."

"Steve and I must just be nervous people. When we were being treated for infertility, we were worried all the time — about test results, side effects, and the lack of control over our lives. I thought the worrying would end with my pregnancy, but it has just shifted focus. In the first trimester we worried about whether the pregnancy might miscarry. Now that I'm in the second trimester, we've begun to worry about what could go wrong with the delivery. Somehow it seems that we don't feel entitled to enjoy this pregnancy until we have a healthy baby in our arms."

"I'm having such fun buying maternity clothes — I can remember my years of infertility when I actually wouldn't even go to the place in the mall where the maternity shop is located. I couldn't bear to see the pregnant women shopping there, knowing that I might never be able to. Now my maternity clothes are a real symbol of my victory over infertility."

"Joe and I are thrilled with how the pregnancy is progressing, so that's a real relief. But we also realize we were so caught up in our infertility treatment that we hadn't fully appreciated some of the challenges parenthood would bring. So now, at the same time that we're feeling so happy, we are looking at our bank account to decide how we can support the additional expenses of a baby, whether we'll both need to work full time, whether our apartment is going to be big enough, and all sorts of other practical questions."

Emotions in the Third Trimester

By the third trimester the focus shifts once again to delivery and parenthood. Unless there have been complications in the pregnancy, the third trimester becomes a time of eager anticipation, with some apprehensions about the delivery. These apprehensions are fueled by your earlier experiences with medical procedures focused on your reproductive health. Since the outcome of some of those procedures was not what you hoped for, you probably still carry with you a heightened sensitivity that the outcome of your baby's delivery carries risks. For now, however, you're focused on keeping healthy in this last trimester, as each week of pregnancy confirms that the baby is developing well.

The energy in earlier months that focused on hopefulness is now channeled in more concrete ways. You and your partner discuss names, make more frequent visits to the obstetrician or midwife, furnish the nursery, attend childbirth classes, read books on delivery and nursing and infant care, select a pediatrician, and make final plans for the trip to the hospital and help at home after the baby's arrival. In many ways, the endless planning of this period is in direct contrast to the feelings of being out of control that characterized your months of infertility.

You now try to structure the most ideal situation as you anticipate parenthood.

Perhaps you can identify with some of these scenarios of the
third trimester and its impact as you and your partner anticipate
the amazing changes that a baby will bring into your lives:

"In some ways I feel as busy as I did during our infertility when
we were rushing from the clinic to the therapist to the drugstore
and trying to fit it all into our work and personal lives. But this
is so much more fun! I love the decisions that we're making —
colors for the nursery, names, which stroller to buy . . . I feel as if
I'm in a dream world and all it will take to complete the dream
is to wake up with our baby in my arms."

"Frankly, as thrilled as I am to be pregnant, I'm finding myself
irritated at the way some of our family members are suddenly
intruding on our lives. When we were infertile, it's like we had
an invisible disease — no one wanted to talk about it or about
how upsetting it was for us. Now that we're expecting and the
pregnancy has progressed to the third trimester, all of a sudden
everyone wants to get in on the act, suggesting names, offering
hand-me-downs, and talking incessantly about their labors and
deliveries. I guess I find it upsetting that it takes a pregnancy for
me to be embraced by my family again."

"This third trimester is a time when my partner Jennifer is anticipating all the legal work involved in preparing to adopt our baby
after it is born. On the one hand, it makes us both angry that
she needs to go through legal steps that no one would require
of a married couple. And certainly the idea that a case worker
will do a home study to evaluate her as an adequate parent is
just downright insulting. But, on the other hand, now that we
are so close to becoming parents, this trimester also is a time

to celebrate with our friends and family who have been so supportive of our decision to become parents."

"During introductions at our first childbirth class, Joan introduced herself as my sister-in-law, and I could see the puzzled looks on the faces of the other couples. I wasn't sure how to present myself as an enthusiastic single mother-to-be and, sure enough, a good number of couples in the class initially assumed that this was an unplanned pregnancy. But I decided to be clear that I had conceived this baby with lots of reproductive assistance, and eventually everyone just included Joan and me in the informal conversation before and after the class. But I do feel that I stand out as a 'different' mother in a group, and I guess I'd better figure out a comfortable way of conveying my happiness at my choice to be a single mother."

"When I was a teenager I did a lot of babysitting, so I have a pretty good idea of how to diaper and burp and soothe crying infants. In spite of his passion about becoming a father, Steve hasn't even held a baby before, let alone become familiar with its daily functions! I've told him that I'm going to need to learn about breast-feeding, but that I know he's perfectly capable of learning how to bathe and change a baby, and these are experiences that I really hope he'll take on to feel closer to the baby. He seems hesitant, but willing to give it a try. He's even agreed to take lessons from my brother, who has volunteered his infant for supervised bathing and diapering!"

"After all the infertility procedures I've undergone, I'm feeling pretty apprehensive about the delivery. So much can go wrong, and my body has never been something I could count on when it comes to making babies. I guess I worry that it may let me down during the delivery too. As much as I like our obstetrician, the whole idea of having a doctor involved again brings back the memories of all the surgeries when I was infertile."

Unanticipated Complications

For women who have pregnancy complications, the earlier feelings of being out of control resurface. Once again you must depend on health-care professionals. Once again you are reminded that your body is not handling its reproductive capacities smoothly. Once again you feel the fear in the pit of your stomach that perhaps, even now, this pregnancy is going to defy your every effort to have a healthy outcome.

Having sustained the pregnancy until the third trimester is a measured victory. Yet, with the fear of premature labor looming, it is possible that your obstetrician has told you to curtail your activity or to be on strict bed rest, either at home or the maternity ward, where your pregnancy can be closely monitored.

The hospital environment forces you to confront the constant reminders of your body's unpredictability, even as you observe with envy the parents on the ward who are learning to care for their newborns. This is a trying time for you and your partner, as you are reminded once again that having a baby is not an experience to take for granted. Whether your bed rest is at home or in the hospital, this forced period of dependency keeps you and your partner from having the kind of mutual pre-parenting experiences that most other couples enjoy. However, with your focus being on day-to-day successes, you are eternally hopeful that the end of this trimester will be a smooth delivery and a healthy baby, as these women's stories demonstrate:

"The minute the doctor ordered me to bed I knew I was going to be robbed of feeling fully joyful about this pregnancy. Now I'm so tuned in to every movement the baby makes, to every twinge of my uterus, and to every fear I could imagine about a premature delivery. Earlier in the pregnancy I had all sorts of things to distract me — now it's just me in this bed feeling funky, unproductive, and obsessed with wanting this pregnancy to be healthy."

"With the doctor saying that I needed to begin my maternity leave two months earlier than I had expected, I'm at loose ends. I sort of feel as if I'm under house arrest, since I can't drive either. Now I appreciate how the structure of work and being involved with the outside world was such a vital part of my life. I was a miserable infertility patient, and I can feel lots of those reactions resurfacing, even when a different doctor is calling the shots. I just have to keep in mind that things are really more hopeful now that I'm pregnant — I just hope the baby stays put until closer to my delivery date."

"Being in the hospital so much earlier than I had expected is tough. I feel guilty about going on maternity leave weeks earlier than I'd planned, and now Tim is left with getting the nursery in order — and I'd really looked forward to doing that with him! With all these worries about the baby's health, there is a part of me that wants to tell him to wait until the baby is born before finishing the nursery — is that morbid or what? But I've had so much sadness with our infertility that these last complications are just another reminder that being pregnant is no guarantee of a healthy baby."

Post-birth Concerns

Pregnancy and a healthy birth represent the dreams that you have nourished throughout your pregnancy. Will any ghosts of infertility lurk in the corners once you have a healthy baby sleeping in the nursery? I will mention a few, not to preoccupy you, but to reassure you that it is normal for these ghosts to float in and out of your consciousness as a new parent:

- *Being overprotective* is both expected and common for previously infertile couples. This baby is especially precious, and you are aware that it may be your only birth child. So it is not surprising that you want to do everything possible to keep it safe and healthy in every way. Just be careful if you find yourself being overly vigilant or reluctant to let your growing child take in new experiences.

- *Being stoic*, which you may have been during your pregnancy as you refused to acknowledge the misery of nausea and fatigue, may resurface. This time your stoicism may kick in as you endure sleep deprivation, the boredom (or hectic aspects) of your daily routine, the lack of down time, and the juggling of your new roles and responsibilities that may not be going as smoothly as you had hoped. Just be aware that it is emotionally healthier for you to communicate your frustrations than to keep them bottled up. Only by letting others know what you need can you make a plan that will reduce your exhaustion or feelings of being overwhelmed.

- *Striving for perfectionism*, whether it is keeping up with the laundry or being ready for your baby's next developmental phase, is a temptation for all parents. Now that your baby is such a significant focus in your life, you want to create the best environment possible. But don't be too hard on yourself (or on your partner) when you must adjust carefully laid plans. Or, more likely, when you lack the time and energy even to plan more than a few hours ahead! Focus on the joys and pleasures of parenthood and partnership, and try to take the ups and downs in stride.

- *Feeling guilty,* which is especially unproductive, can be triggered by a variety of circumstances: ambivalence about parenthood, fatigue, difficulty juggling family responsibilities smoothly, challenges of renegotiating familiar relationships, doubt about day-care arrangements, and myriad other day-to-day irritations. If you can, try to talk to other new mothers about their experiences with parenthood. You'll find some guilt is universal, but some new mothers will carry fewer emotional burdens than others, and their perspectives may be useful to consider as you realign your priorities. After all, parenthood is an evolving process, and being open to new ways of coping is a real plus.

- *Experiencing depression,* possibly a familiar feeling from infertile days, may now be related to the changes in your hormones following your delivery. It may be exacerbated by fatigue, the feeling that your body will never get its shape back, the monotony of changing diapers, frequent feedings, and a squalling infant. For most women, depression passes as they begin to establish a routine that enables them to get more rest and more participation from their partner. However, if you are among the women whose depression does not lift, or if you have thoughts of doing harm to yourself or to your baby, you may be experiencing *postpartum depression.* If so, it is time to share this information with your ob-gyn and identify a mental health professional who can immediately assess how best to help you. If you are not sure how to begin this process, you can contact your community's mental health society. Other sources include the social worker at the hospital where you delivered your baby, your ob-gyn, your clergy, or the Resources section at the end of this book. The sooner you reach out for help, the more quickly you will experience relief from the weight of this depression.

Therapeutic Tips

Once you have a positive pregnancy test, you know how precious this pregnancy is. As you try to balance your feelings of apprehension and hope, you are keenly aware that your infertility continues to influence the ways you and your partner view this pregnancy and your preparation for your new roles as parents. Pregnancy books are not likely to include any of the tips below, which are especially timely for you as you hope for a healthy pregnancy and safe delivery:

• You may be tempted to stop going to your support group or seeing your counselor once you hear the welcome news of a positive pregnancy test. However, don't be so hasty to take up membership in The Club that you distance yourself prematurely from your support system! During this pregnancy you are likely to experience periodic feelings of anxiety that can be best assuaged by empathic friends or a familiar therapist who has traveled the infertility pathway with you. If your infertility support group does not allow pregnant couples, see whether your infertility clinic or a nearby chapter of the Infertility Awareness Association of Canada (IAAC) or RESOLVE has a support group that feels right for you. You may not need to meet with your therapist as frequently as during your infertile months, but it is a good idea to schedule regular meetings to check in — you'll be surprised at how infertility has conditioned you to see this pregnancy uniquely.

• You may be trying to decide with your partner how soon to share the news of your pregnancy. Although you may be tempted to wait until after the first trimester, when the risk of a miscarriage diminishes, it is important to ask yourselves why you are waiting. Most couples wait because they fear a miscarriage or a negative outcome of prenatal testing. But if (heaven forbid) that happens, won't you want to gather around you the love and support of family and friends who know how much this pregnancy has meant to you? An early loss, even before you look pregnant, is still a very real loss to mourn, and you absolutely deserve to have the support of loved ones at such a difficult emotional time. How much information to disclose is up to you, but do be aware that people who love you can more easily offer their comfort and support if they have known about the pregnancy from the earliest weeks.

• You are undoubtedly relishing the fun experiences in which you could not indulge during your months or years of trying to conceive: buying maternity clothes, looking at baby furniture, knitting or crocheting blankets or baby garments. But also unspoken during those childless years were some practical decisions that you and your partner now need to discuss: finances, child-care arrangements, chores, and parenting responsibilities. Take your time, but be aware that enlarging your family means changes to physical space, bank accounts, leisure time, family responsibilities, and work-life balance (although the word *balance* may disappear from your vocabulary for months at a time!). The more you agree on these practical issues before the baby's birth, the easier it will be to renegotiate new arrangements as the baby grows.

• You and your partner may consider setting boundaries with families and loved ones. This will differ with every family. Single parents and lesbians will very likely create families from loved ones and close friends who may not be blood relatives. Married couples will also need to decide how to negotiate relationships with existing family members, who often feel especially entitled to offer advice, make demands, and be involved in your life now that you, too, are parents. Only you know the parties involved, with their unique strengths and limitations. The guiding considerations to keep in mind are whether the preferences of family are contributing to your strengths as partners and parents; whether they are in the best interest of the health and safety of your child; and whether they allow for reciprocity in a comfortable way across the generations. Often the reactions and behaviors of family members during your difficult years of trying to conceive have left their mark, either positive or negative. Pay attention to their behaviors now to see how your new relationship might evolve as you take on your roles as parents.

You and your partner are entering uncharted territory as parents, which can be both exciting and daunting. You both may have idealized this period of your lives as you looked with anticipation to having your dreams fulfilled. The reality of disrupted sleep, piles of laundry, a curtailed social life, and a to-do list that never ends will require cooperation and humor from both of you. If you are a single parent, now is the time to draw on the goodwill of relatives, friends, and neighbors to let them know how they can provide much-needed support — there is nothing like a new baby to bring out solicitous offers of help! In the midst of it all, you will have no difficulty recalling the much darker days as you were trying to conceive, which make most challenges of new parenthood pale by comparison! So get as much rest as you can, share the errands, be patient with yourself, breathe deeply, and relish how the meaning of family has taken on new and unexpected dimensions.

Ten

Ending Treatment:
When Enough Is Enough

The decision to let go of your quest for a birth child comes in stages, in ebbs and flows of emotion that are laced with grief and ambivalence. On the one hand is the tremendous amount of energy you have devoted to overcoming your infertility. This energy has consumed you, altered your relationships, diminished your financial resources, put your life on hold, and ultimately changed the person you are and the way you view the world. On the other hand, at the very time you have been investing energy in overcoming your infertility, you have yearned for some stability, predictability, and control over your life and the decisions that you face. You ask yourself how much longer you can keep this up, and wonder about other options besides being a birth parent that could bring you happiness. If you let go of your dream child, could you live happily in a world full of infants, children, and pregnant women?

Many couples wish that their physicians would simply tell them there is no hope and, indeed, some physicians do. But far more common are the messages that "one more try," "another approach," or "a few more cycles" might lead to a healthy pregnancy, and it is in the midst of these seductive messages that couples realize they are the ones who ultimately will need to call a halt. At a time when medical advances once seemed so promising, what factors will you consider as you make the decision to stop infertility treatment? In this chapter, I will explore some of these practical factors that you and your partner will need to discuss, including finances, time disruptions, clinic accessibility, work performance, statistical odds, and emotional issues.

Finances

Most individuals begin diagnosis and treatment full of hope. But it isn't long before the costly realities become a factor in how long you believe you can continue treatment. These realities include limits of insurance coverage, time away from work, and housing accommodations if your clinic is in a distant city. It isn't only that your bank account is depleted — you may also need to anticipate costs associated with later choices to pursue adoption or surrogacy. You may want to consider putting a limit on how low you are willing to draw your savings account, so that if you do not become pregnant you still will have some savings set aside to pursue other options.

"We have spent our life's savings trying to have a baby. The idea of giving up now makes me feel as if we've just thrown all that money, time, and hope down the drain — and all for what? For the sadness of not being a parent?"

"Frankly, we just don't have any more money that we can devote to this. We have no savings, we've borrowed from both sets of parents, and if we continue at this rate we'll be in hock up to our ears. If the doctors could offer any encouragement I might be willing to continue, but with no optimism from them that I can get pregnant, we just have to cut our losses."

"Even though we've been lucky that our insurance has covered a number of procedures, it won't continue to finance our treatments indefinitely or even to be a resource if we move into a more high-tech set of treatments. And, since our clinic is very far away, we have to bear the expenses of hotel costs and time lost from work, and those costs are beginning to mount up."

"We sat down the other night to talk about our bank account. Jim asked whether I wanted to spend thousands of dollars on treatments with no promises of success or whether we might consider taking the money we have left and pursuing adoption, which he thinks will offer more possibilities of bringing a child into our family."

Time Disruptions

The loss of other opportunities while you pursue treatment feels like a dark cloud hanging over you. Remembering that you began infertility treatment with high hopes, it is important to re-evaluate those hopes and other life goals every six months or so. Your physician, a support group, or a counselor can help you think through whether (or for how long) you want to sacrifice your other goals to the quest for a pregnancy.

"You know, the money has been a very concrete loss in all of this. But another loss has been my devoting three years of my life to trying to conquer infertility, when I could have been using those years to get more education, to get ahead in a career, or just to enjoy life. I feel like I've wasted this time and I'll never get it back."

"We have given years to this quest for parenthood. When we began, we were thinking in terms of months. This period of sadness in our life together is becoming too long."

"I haven't taken a vacation in three years, because we need to be near the clinic for various procedures and treatments, and I haven't wanted to lose so much as a month. I can't imagine trying to enjoy myself on vacation, while wondering the whole time if this might have been the month I could have conceived."

Clinic Accessibility

Access to quality clinic services may involve a lengthy and costly commute. Ask the counselor at your clinic what their other patients do to reduce the cost and disruption of a commute. Explore whether some of your tests and blood draws can be performed locally and the results faxed to the clinic. If you are in a support group, ask its members if they have found creative solutions to this dilemma. In some cases you may be able to find a nearby reproductive endocrinologist or urologist in private practice who could perform most of the diagnostic and treatment interventions that you need. If so, consider working with a reproductive specialist whose office is much more accessible than your clinic.

"Even though my partner and I live near a good infertility clinic in the US, we are not eligible for services there because they insist their patients be married. As lesbians we don't have that option where we live. As much as I'd like to challenge the clinic's policy as discriminatory, I've decided to put my energies into a much longer commute to a different clinic. But it is exhausting, time consuming, and expensive to go that extra distance."

"The closest clinic to our home is about a three-hour drive. We decided that I'll simply rent a little apartment in that city and stay there whenever I need to, since I'm the one who has to undergo the most time-consuming procedures. We're lucky that money isn't a big issue. But the separation from Tom, especially while I'm waiting for test results, is just agonizing."

"We have a farm, and whenever we both need to travel to the clinic, which is 300 miles away, it means that we need to hire people to do the farm work — after all, the cows need to be milked whether it's convenient for us or not! But all of this travel to a high-quality clinic is a real disruption and also a big expense."

Work Performance

Pride in your work may be especially significant when you are feeling unproductive in your efforts to become pregnant. You will not know the medical demands on your time until you have been in treatment for some time. Initially you may have communicated to your supervisor and coworkers what you believed would be the impact of your periodic absences. But, as that changes, it is relevant to offer some updated information about why your schedule must adapt to medical routines. You have a few choices: asking to be assigned a workload that you believe is flexible enough for you to manage (perhaps including some work from a distance), putting an "end point" to your treatments, and deciding to explore other options for parenthood that are not as work-disruptive, or leaving (permanently or with a sabbatical) your current place of employment, if you can afford to, so that the stress of your infertility is not compounded by the stress of performing below par in the workplace.

"I cannot tell you how awful it is to choose between having good continuity in my work at the office and fitting in the clinic appointments. I love my work, and doing less than my best makes me feel that I could lose my professional life just as I'm having to accept that I may never get pregnant."

"Although we were overjoyed to find a clinic within a two hour drive that offers infertility treatment, we had no real understanding of what it would mean to have to go there regularly. My absences, some of which are more than just a day when we figure in the travel time, are affecting the quality of my work at the office. And I feel guilty to have my coworkers picking up the work I'm not there to do."

Statistical Odds or a Poor Medical Prognosis

The scenarios in this section are heartbreaking, but they also are a reminder that not everyone is going to be a promising patient for infertility treatment. If you know that your statistics are not hopeful, it is important to combine consultation with your physician and counseling with a therapist as ways of bringing together information and insight about why you are continuing with infertility treatment when the odds are against success.

"When I began treatment I was in my late thirties. Now I am in my early forties, and even if I'm able to conceive, I worry about the age of my eggs and whether or not I could have a healthy baby. Frankly, I don't think I could bear a miscarriage, and the possibility that there might be a problematic prenatal diagnosis is more than I can contemplate."

"After five years of treatment with every procedure my doctor could offer, I still haven't had even one pregnancy. It seems to me, my husband, and the doctor that trying longer isn't likely to lead to a healthy pregnancy."

"Although my infertility treatment has resulted in four pregnancies, it has also resulted in four miscarriages. No one knows why I am unable to have a healthy pregnancy, but the odds of another pregnancy being successful are not promising."

Emotional Issues

In addition to the rational issues, there are also the emotional issues that are part of any decision to discontinue treatment. Couples may be influenced by their beliefs about genetic continuity; by the woman's visceral yearning for pregnancy, childbirth, and breast-feeding; by issues of "success"; or by a wish not to confront the necessary mourning that will accompany the end of a medical quest for a birth child.

Genetic continuity may be important to one or both partners, and it also may be an issue for parents or in-laws:

"In my family we've always made a big deal of family connections. Whether it has been the jokes about who resembles whom, or the admiration for talents that appear in each generation, there's no question that family genes are important to us."

"My fantasy baby is a mix of Alan's red hair and freckles and my slim build and musical talent. I know it's possible that we could give birth to a chubby, tone-deaf brunette, but even in a baby who's different from what I imagine, I would love to see some genetic resemblances."

"My father-in-law has been so sad about our infertility. And he is clear that Mitch, as his only child, is the person in the family that will bring the next generation into this world. Accepting an adopted grandchild would be very difficult for him. And when the doctors asked Mitch and me how we felt about using donor sperm, we both ended up discussing his father's attitudes."

"Both sides of our family place a premium on being bright and going to college. I know that it is possible that we could have a birth child who is not college material, but I think I could accept that more easily if I knew we both had given him our genes and it just didn't work out. To accept a baby into our lives without those genes would cause us to blame ourselves if that child didn't end up being bright and inquisitive."

Many women associate parenthood with the joys of seeing their bodies change to nourish a pregnancy, to deliver a healthy baby, and to breast-feed an infant:

"Ending infertility treatment is the end of my dream of being pregnant. Everyone I see around me is pregnant, and it seems so unfair to be deprived of that joyful nine months. After all these years of infertility, I just wanted to present myself pregnant to the world and watch my belly grow and feel little baby kicks!"

"When I have imagined having a baby, I have imagined showing pictures in our family scrapbook of me growing more and more pregnant, of me holding a baby in the delivery room, and of me nursing the little darling. The idea that I'll never have any of these experiences is really emotional for me."

"After all this time of having my body be the focus of infertility treatments, I kept holding out the hope that the ultimate reward would be a baby growing inside me. I wouldn't mind the morning sickness or the stretch marks. The loss of this experience is immeasurable."

"There's something magical to me about giving birth. In spite of my worry about the pain, I found myself fantasizing about the magic of delivering a baby into this world, nursing it, and cuddling it. It's just tragic that my body has betrayed me and denied me this experience. Giving up on treatment means I can never have this special bond with a baby."

For women who take joy in successes, who are competitive, or who believe that hard work is rewarded, the thought of stopping treatment can feel like failing. For someone with that perspective, infertility has been perceived as a barrier to be overcome, and the incapacity to do so can be bitter and can contribute to ambivalence about ending treatment:

"At heart I'm a pretty competitive person. When I put my mind to something, I usually get what I want. My attitude is that if I try my best, I should be able to achieve my goal. But infertility has been a real wake-up call. This is one game I finally have to admit I'm not going to win. Not by sheer determination, not by seeking out the best doctors, not by tolerating the most awful side effects, not even by praying. I guess it's a comfort to know that I've done all I can do, but the question is still out there: what if I had hung on just a couple of months longer?"

"For my whole life I've been admired and complimented for the successes I've had. I've worked for every one of them and I've always believed that hard work is rewarded. Now, when a baby is really the only thing I want, I feel like a miserable failure. It seems that there's nothing I can do to have the one success that matters more than all of the others combined."

The incapacity to experience a healthy pregnancy despite medical treatment calls forth a range of emotions. Every woman is familiar with the sadness, the disappointment, the rage, the frustration, and the helplessness brought on by infertility. For some women it is easier to experience those emotions month after month than to confront the feelings of loss that accompany the decision to end treatment:

"I think I held off ending my infertility treatments until now because if I'm not going to be a mother, I really don't see a future for myself. Ever since we've been married my view of my future has included children. In my wildest nightmares, I never envisioned that infertility would take me so far off track. So now that I'm letting go of my dreams of being a birth mother, it's pretty scary to see this big world looming out in front of me."

"I am so worn out emotionally from the mood swings, from the sadness of getting my period month after month, and from the realization that I am running out of options. But I feel as if giving up now would just be another huge emotional burden to bear — it feels somehow more hopeful to keep on trying, even though I know there's so little chance."

"Pursuing infertility treatment has been a huge project, complete with research, scheduling, and learning about procedures and results. It has kept me completely preoccupied. Frankly, I'm exhausted and I'm upset at the amount of energy I had to devote to something that had no joyful outcome. If we decide to adopt, I don't know if I'll have the energy to begin all over again with the research, the paperwork, and the interminable waiting."

"By ending my treatments, I feel as if I'm moving from having very few choices to suddenly having too many choices. I can't choose to be a birth mother, which is what I really want. But once I accept that that door is closed, I feel as if I'm in a corridor of lots of other doors of life choices. The challenge is going to be what choices can make Cory and me happy."

Letting Go

Letting go inevitably involves mourning. You will mourn the dream child that you cannot give birth to, and you will relinquish the dreams of any other children you had hoped would complete your family. You will mourn the loss of your role as a birth mother and all of the hopes you associate with this role: a joyful pregnancy, an uncomplicated labor, a victorious delivery, peaceful breast-feeding, and the rewards and challenges of parenting. Unless you decide to pursue other ways of building your family, you will mourn the loss of those things you had anticipated sharing with your partner: parenting, rejoicing in your child's successes, enjoying family leisure and vacations through a child's eyes, and planning for a child-centered future. And, at some level, you will mourn that you are the last generation. That when you and your partner die no one will carry on the family genes, the family stories, the family jokes, and whatever legacy you would have shared with a birth child.

This is a lot to mourn. Making the decision to stop infertility treatments can feel like several deaths. And in North American culture, where even real death is but briefly ritualized, there is no ritual for accepting your lifelong infertility and all the losses it involves. As you are well aware, only people who have experienced infertility can appreciate how much pain and sorrow are involved in the unsuccessful pursuit of a healthy pregnancy. And, sympathetic as loved ones may be about your decision to let go, they also are likely to be relieved that now you can get on with your life. Women who decide to let go will confront the situation in different ways:

"My mother was so relieved when we told her that we were giving up on medical treatments. 'Now you can get your life back,' she said to me. But how do you just walk away from the dreams of a baby who will never come to life? How do you take joy in going to work every day when you still sit down at the family dinner table with just one other person? How do you fill your life with activities that have meaning?"

"After we decided not to pursue treatment any longer, I took some vacation time and gathered up all the reminders of our baby who was not to be: an empty baby scrapbook, a baby name book, a couple of cute maternity dresses, and some children's books I had picked up at a library sale. One of our neighbors just announced that she is due in six months, so I asked her if she wanted them, and she was thrilled. I needed to give them a good home, since I took so much care in choosing them."

"Jake never had been as emotionally attached as I was to the hope of a baby. All along he was more concerned with my mood swings, with my feelings of desperation, and with my fixation that we *had* to have a baby. So when the doctors made it clear that they had run out of options, I think Jake was relieved that we could get our lives back. But it was really important for me to tell him that I needed his emotional support as I came to terms with the knowledge that I would never become pregnant or bear our child. He would have preferred to distract me from my sadness, but once I made it clear that I needed time to heal emotionally, he took his signals from me."

"As much as I maintained that the sadness of infertility was greater for me than it was for my husband, I think this was just because I couldn't bear his grief on top of my own. When we decided that there really was no point in continuing treatment, we talked a lot about what that decision meant for each of us. Our parents and siblings haven't been especially understanding during this time, but our pastor has been. We asked if he would pray with us to help us let go of our baby dreams and open our hearts to the new possibilities that life has to offer. He was eloquent and caring. We are so fortunate to have been able to lean on him, both during our years of treatment and especially as we ended that part of our lives."

"When my therapist asked me what was the hardest part of discontinuing treatment, I said that I just hadn't found a way to put my dream child, Debbie, to rest. I still could picture her, and I still cherished her in my dreams, although I'd stopped talking to her in my imagination. My therapist suggested that we create a small ceremony where I could put Debbie to rest. So that's what we did. We decided to have the ceremony in a nearby meadow where we have taken so many walks and talked about our hopes of getting pregnant. We invited our parents and a few very close friends. We read some poetry, then Stan and I read the letters we each had composed to our dream baby, then we attached the letters to a helium balloon and launched it off into the sky. I think, for us, this was the ideal way to bring closure so we could move on."

Moving On

As you give up the dream of a birth child, you also are giving up the entire future that was associated with the birth of your baby. It can feel as if you have a gaping hole where before there had been hopes and dreams. So one challenge is how to make new dreams.

Another challenge is how to come to terms with what infertility now means in your life. There is an identity in trying to conceive, and without that preoccupation you may feel empty. Previously your infertility had been a rallying cry to health professionals, to sympathetic loved ones, to people in Internet chat rooms, members of support groups, and counselors. But now that you are no longer pursuing medical treatment, some people will assume that you have put your infertility behind you. Your challenge will be how to integrate infertility into who you are becoming in the months and years ahead as you attempt to move on:

"It's a funny thing. When I decided to end treatment, I thought that I would feel relief at not needing to subject myself to the disruptions, the side effects, and the discouraging test results. But as I was saying my goodbyes and offering thanks to the clinic staff and to the doctor who has seen us through three years of unsuccessful treatment, I also was struck with how much I would miss their caring, their encouragement, and their concern. These were special relationships. I know they wanted very much for me to leave the clinic with a pregnancy and to return with a baby for them to fuss over."

"My therapist and I are still discussing whether we have work to do. Even though she offered support and insight as I brought closure to my dreams of being a birth mother, and even though she was integral to helping Joe and me process the pros and cons of adoption, I'm not sure I want to continue in therapy now that we've decided to adopt. Ending therapy and pursuing adoption are my ways of asserting that we are moving down a new path with more hope and less grief than the infertility treatments. I think I'd like to try it on my own, but it's good to know that she will be there if I need her support."

"When I told the members of my support group that Kelly and I had decided to withdraw from treatment, I was really touched with the warmth of responses that they offered. Several of them who are pursuing adoption offered to share their materials with us if we decided to adopt. Others said that they would be glad for us to stay in the support group as long as we needed to. That was a real comfort, because they know me so well, and they can understand what this decision represents for me after five years of treatment. These folks are dear friends, and I didn't want to lose their friendship at the very time I was struggling with giving up one of my life dreams."

However you come to the decision to discontinue infertility treatment, you will also need to come to terms with your own future and the role that a child can play in it. Has adoption become more attractive? Have you decided to weigh the risks of having a surrogate bear your child? Does child-free living seem more possible now? In the next chapter I will examine the various options that many people consider after ending infertility treatment.

Therapeutic Tips

As you read this chapter, you are likely to realize that you have been preparing yourself for these issues for some time. As efforts to become pregnant have consumed more and more time, energy, money, and stamina, questions have crept into your mind; "Will I spend my life trying to have a baby?" and "What if nothing works?" and "How much longer can I keep my life on hold?" are just a few. Now, as you contemplate what it will mean to close this door, here are some tips to help you in this part of your journey:

• Take a gradual approach to your decision to end treatment. Since it is very likely that you and your partner are not on the same psychological page, one goal is to come closer together in discussing the factors that influence your decisions. You can begin this process by making a list of the factors identified in this chapter and weighing with your partner whether or how much longer to continue treatment.

• Have a straightforward discussion with your infertility specialist about the pros and cons of continuing treatment. Remember, however, that this physician is weighing your information from a medical perspective, and you need to consider carefully the other factors in your life that are affected by continuing treatment.

• Consider setting some limits for yourselves: 1) a date in the future when you will end treatment if you have not become pregnant; 2) a bank account balance below which you will not withdraw money for treatment; and 3) a date by which another important decision (grad school, new job application, down payment on a home) must be made that conflicts with your capacity to continue treatment, and validates your wish to move forward with your lives.

- Gather information from others in your support group who are deciding whether to end treatment, from adoptive parents, or from child-free individuals and couples about the process they used to reach their decisions about ending treatment and moving forward. Ask if they would do anything differently if they had it to do over again. Ask if they had support in making their decision, and ask who supported them. This will ease you a little closer to the reality of ending treatment while opening doors to new information and to choices that are still available to you.

- Consider seeking the assistance of a counselor who can help you weigh alternatives and make decisions. Although the decision you reach *is* a significant turning point in your hopes of becoming a parent, the way in which you get to that point is a *process*, which requires time, discussion, and careful consideration. Since this process may cause tension in your relationship with your partner, it can be very helpful to have a counselor on board to attend to the feelings generated, as well as to provide input to the concrete decisions you are weighing.

Although you ultimately will see ending treatment as closing a door, remember that being in treatment has taught you and your partner some things about yourselves, your resilience, your priorities, and your relationship. This knowledge will hopefully serve as a good foundation upon which you can move forward with future discussions and decisions. Keep in mind the potential importance of having support in this process, whether from loved ones, professionals, or other people who, like yourselves, have decided to open different doors on the journey to parenthood or to child-free living.

Eleven

Different Dreams: *Opening New Doors to Life*

Individuals and couples who decide to discontinue infertility treatment have a range of new emotional and practical directions to pursue. Ending treatment is itself a monumental decision, one that plunges you into a morass of uncertainty and a wellspring of possibilities. And those possibilities will be influenced by everything from your finances and your age to the reactions of your extended family and the supportiveness of your community. In this chapter you will hear from couples who are weighing the options that are available once they discontinue their efforts to become pregnant: adoption, surrogacy, or living child free. (At the end of this book is a list of resources that you may want to consult for more information about these options.)

Adoption

Adoption, the preferred next step for infertile couples, has changed dramatically over the past 50 years. One major change has been a result of the availability of birth control and abortion.

Not only have the rates of unplanned pregnancies declined in Canada and the US, but also the pool of infants available for adoption has changed. Now, with relatively small numbers of healthy Caucasian infants being placed with adoptive parents, prospective parents are identifying larger numbers of non-Caucasian babies, older children, sibling groups, and children with special needs.

In the past three decades there has been a surge of international adoptions from Asia, Latin America, Africa, and eastern Europe. The number of children adopted internationally by US citizens has increased 20-fold over 30 years. This poses the challenge for many parents of how to help their child feel connected to the culture of his or her ethnicity or country of birth, about which the parents themselves may know relatively little. It poses the additional consideration of the extent to which the parents' community offers a hospitable environment for children of color, children with special needs, and adopted children in general. Fees for international adoption are comparable to a domestic placement, generally in the range of $15,000–$40,000. When children with special needs are adopted, there may be public agency funds available to cover the costs of counseling, academic assistance, and medical help. International waiting times vary, ranging from six months to two years, a time period that is shorter than for a domestic agency adoption.

There also has been a shift in how individuals and couples with infertility find potential children. Those interested in adopting foster children or children with special needs are most likely to begin with the public agency in their community responsible for such placements. Others place advertisements in newspapers (particularly in university communities) in the hope that a young pregnant woman may consider an offer to adopt her baby; some work with lawyers specializing in adoption to get advice about the most efficient way to locate a potential birth mother; and some look for adoption information using the Internet.

In fact, the Internet has opened up a range of opportunities for prospective adoptive parents: participating in online bulletin boards or chat rooms can provide information, answer questions, help to refine decisions, and offer a receptive audience for hopes, dreams, joys, and frustrations. Adoption agencies also use the Internet to post information on families who have completed their home studies and are now hoping to locate a pregnant woman or new mother who is considering making a plan for her baby's adoption.

Individuals who have used the Internet during their months and years of infertility may consider it a useful resource; however, beginning anew in the area of adoption can easily lead to information overload. In addition, some of the information posted on Web sites is outdated, inaccurate, misleading, or fraudulent, and some of the people who offer themselves online as adoption facilitators use pressure tactics that play upon the desperation of prospective adoptive parents. So while browsing the Web, be an educated consumer and steer clear of those sites that promise quick results with minimum cost or involvement. The best Web sites are those that offer information on how to think about and prepare for adoption, adoption laws, precautions to take, and resources on adoption from beginning to end. (You will find helpful information in the Resources section at the end of this book, where I list Web sites on general adoption, international adoption, interracial adoption, and special needs adoption.)

Before you decide whether adoption is the way to pursue your dream of becoming a parent, it is important to confront some of the myths about adoption:

- *Once you adopt, you'll relax and become pregnant.* Wrong! Adoption is not a cure for infertility. In fact, it is healthy to have resolved your dreams for a birth child before embarking on the search for a child to adopt so that you can devote your full emotional energy to this new challenge. In truth, about 5 percent of women who discontinue infertility treatment become pregnant, whether or not they have pursued adoption.

- *Adoption is an event, rather than a process.* Wrong! Although the event of the adoption itself is a time for celebration, most adoptive parents find that over time the unique identity of their adopted child requires special concern and consideration at different stages of the adoption process.

- *If you're a good parent to your adopted child, he or she will have no interest in learning about his or her birth family.* Wrong! In fact, many adopted children will be curious and interested in learning more about their birth families. Adolescence and young adulthood are stages when this need may feel most compelling (and national resources are available to assist them in their search). A search for the birth parents doesn't mean that the adopted child is rejecting her adoptive family or feeling unloved by them; it is an expression of the adoptee's need to know where she came from, and perhaps why a plan was made for her adoption in the first place.

Next, you will want to examine the many choices that exist for prospective adoptive parents. Some of these choices involve the following factors:

- **Resources:** your financial position, possible time out of the country if you are pursuing an international adoption, the amount of time you are prepared to invest in the adoption;

- **Risks:** possibility that the birth mother may change her mind or that the birth father may want custody, the concern about prenatal care or nutrition of the birth mother during her pregnancy, the impact on the child of months or years spent in an orphanage or in foster care, the lack of trustworthy medical records on the child's growth and development;

- **Type of child or children:** infant, toddler, older child, child with special needs, sibling group;

- **Geography:** country you are considering (where prospective adoptive parents may be told they are ineligible if, for example, they are over a certain age, have specific health problems, are in a same sex relationship, or have had more than one marriage), the laws of certain states (declaring it illegal for unmarried or same sex couples in the US to be adoptive parents), comfort level adopting a child from outside North America or from a different racial or ethnic group; and

- **Privacy:** open or closed adoption.

These choices are challenging at many levels. They require that you confront your biases, examine what kind of child you could love, accept a certain loss of control, decide how open you want family boundaries to be, and imagine how much your own family will need to change to give your new child a welcoming and supportive home. Depending upon your answers, you may decide that you need to give more thought to adoption, that adoption is right for you, or that the risks or difficulties are too much and you will not pursue adoption:

"Although our friends and relatives have been urging us to consider adoption for months now, we realize they mostly want us to move on with our lives after being treated for infertility for so many years. When Ed and I began to discuss what we wanted in our lives if we couldn't have a birth child, we realized that adoption didn't fill either of us with hope. Both of us have been so invested in how our baby would look like us, how it will carry on the family genes through the next generation, and how important pregnancy and nursing are to me. Frankly, neither of us can see ourselves becoming emotionally attached as parents to a child of a different race or ethnicity. And I also know we would worry about whether a birth mother had eaten well during her pregnancy and received the best prenatal care. I guess we are pretty clear that having a birth child is the only way that we want to become parents. So since that isn't an option, and adoption just doesn't feel right, we're going to need to do some hard thinking about next steps in our lives."

"We live in a pretty small rural community where a few couples have adopted their children. All of these have been international adoptions, so these children stand out in our mostly Caucasian town. I wondered how the adoptive parents have handled this issue with their children, so I decided to talk with a few of the mothers who go to our church about my interest in adopting. All of the mothers were very welcoming — that's the bond that infertility can provide, I guess. All of them were glad they had pursued international adoptions, partly because they moved relatively quickly and partly because they worked with organizations that had helped them cut through all the red tape. But all of them said that their children spoke of feeling 'different.' The kids get a lot of questions from their classmates, and all mothers spoke of questions they initially heard from curious people in the grocery store or on the playground. The mothers are pretty philosophical about this, but John and I are really not sure that we want to bring a child into our community who will be made to feel different because of facial features or skin color. This is where both of us grew up, and we don't want to move away, but it is not a community that I believe would support us as an adoptive family. The hard truth is that I think we will need to find a Caucasian baby or to find another way to involve children in our lives."

"When I think about adoption, one of the things that worries me most is we may find a pregnant woman who is willing for us to pay her medical bills during her pregnancy, but who changes her mind once she gives birth. I just don't believe that after my own three miscarriages I could possibly endure losing another baby."

"When I mentioned the possibility of adoption to my parents, it was clear they were less than thrilled. They have provided emotional and financial support to us during our infertility treatments, and they very much want me to be pregnant with their grandchild. A few weeks after our initial conversation, I asked my mother what she had against adoption. She said that she and my father didn't think they could love an adopted baby as much as 'a grandbaby of our own,' and she was worried that Sam and I might be making a serious mistake by considering adoption. I asked whether she believed Sam and I would be happy if we couldn't be parents. That stopped her cold, and I realized that she and my father believe that if we just keep on trying I will get pregnant. So Sam and I sat down with both of them and reviewed what our doctors had concluded — namely that my chances of having a healthy pregnancy are slim and that I'm not getting any younger (and my eggs aren't getting any healthier). We told them that we're not going to rush into this, but that we'd like to share with them the books and articles we can find on adoption. It was a lot to say all at once, but they seem to be more willing to talk about adoption now."

"Adoption has always seemed 'second best' to me. The few adopted kids I knew as a child were not very happy kids, and I guess that has always made me wonder if there would be a cloud hanging over the head of any child we might adopt. Since several members of our infertility support group have adopted, Jay and I decided to talk with them about how they decided it was right for them. I think it is fair to say that all of the couples were enthusiastic about their decision to adopt. They all spoke of how they have talked with their kids from an early age about their adoptions, and several of the parents have encountered insensitive remarks from other adults, but on the whole these parents are real advocates of adoption. They encouraged Jay and me to go to a regional infertility conference where there will be a panel of adoptive parents, so that's next on our list of trying to learn from people who have been in our shoes and who have chosen adoption after infertility."

"Fred and I initially did not believe we could consider adopting a child. Having a pregnancy was so important to me that we only focused on how to accomplish that. Gradually, as it became clearer and clearer that I couldn't get pregnant, we began to talk about adoption. We didn't know any couples our age who had adopted, so we had no one who could relate to our ambivalence. Finally, I said to Fred that we should set a date and if I weren't pregnant by then, we would begin to look into what would be involved with adoption. That date was several months ago. Although we agreed to continue at the clinic for a few more cycles, now our energy is going into reading everything we can get our hands on about adoption. It's kind of scary, but it also seems as if we're much more willing to consider it than we were even a year ago."

"As lesbians, my partner and I are constantly confronting discrimination. We were both very open to adoption, so that's where we turned our energy after ending infertility treatment. Since we have many gay and lesbian friends who are adoptive parents, we actually were unprepared to learn that certain countries would not consider us as applicants for international adoption. For a while I even considered presenting myself as a single straight woman, but our lawyer friends told us that could seriously jeopardize the success of an adoption if anyone discovered that I were lying. So, with some help from our friends, we have found an agency that is comfortable working with gays and lesbians. I am still feeling apprehensive at the prospect of the home study, which I know will feel intrusive, but we want so much to be parents that I know I'll keep that as my main focus."

"Once Ron and I decided we would pursue adoption, we found ourselves intrigued by the possibility of an open adoption. I'm someone who is more concerned with my baby feeling loved than I am with my baby believing that she just has one mother and I'm that person. The idea that we could keep the lines of communication open with the birth mother made me feel as if we would be doing the right thing for her, for the baby, and for us. Of course, Ron and I felt as if this will only work with a birth mother who is mature enough to have her own support system and her own life apart from being a parent. So right now that is where we're headed. I'm looking forward to meeting other adoptive parents who have pursued open adoption so I can learn its pitfalls and rewards."

"In retrospect, I realize that in spite of my months of infertility treatment, I actually want to have a baby more than to give birth to a baby. The idea of morning sickness and stretch marks never appealed to me, and I know I would have chosen not to nurse a baby after it was born. So when Barry and I were discussing how much longer to pursue medical treatment, we both realized that adoption was a really viable alternative for us. Both of us traveled extensively to developing countries in our early twenties, and we have a real love for several South American countries where we lived. I would be thrilled to adopt from any one of those countries and to share with the child our fascination with the culture and the hospitality we experienced. Adopting internationally could open up opportunities to renew our early explorations of our baby's birth country."

"When I stop to consider the number of babies languishing in orphanages around the world, and when I consider how much Joe and I have to give a baby, both emotionally and materially, it makes complete sense to open our hearts and adopt. I know I'm apprehensive about the health of a baby whose mother may not have received good nutrition during pregnancy, and who may not have received much stimulation in an orphanage. But I also know that babies can be resilient. And since one of my siblings had several physical disabilities, I understand the adjustments required on the part of parents. Joe and I have so much love to give each other that I just know we would find a way of adapting even if the child we adopt has special needs."

"We have an adopted daughter who is now three years old. In the past year, Jeff and I have been exploring adopting a second baby. To our utter amazement, we learned last week that I am pregnant! Instead of being filled with joy, I found myself fearful that our daughter, Teresa, would wonder whether we love her sibling more because that baby is our birth child. For about a day I actually contemplated terminating the pregnancy and proceeding with our second adoption. Jeff and I immediately booked an appointment with the therapist we had seen years ago before we adopted Teresa. Fortunately she knows us well from our years of infertility, so she was able to help us sort out issues of expectable sibling rivalry, worries about the viability of the pregnancy, how to help Teresa feel important as the 'big sister,' and how to stretch our lives to make time for two children. So, for me, adoption would have been emotionally easier, but now I have a better perspective on how to keep my anxieties in check."

"For many years I believed that I would meet someone with whom I would share my life. When that never happened, I decided not to give up on my dream of being a parent. Having experienced premature menopause, I saw adoption as a real opportunity to share my life with a child. In the midst of all the paperwork, I realized that this baby deserved to have more people in its life than one enthusiastic mother, so I began a careful inventory of my siblings, friends, neighbors, and relatives to see who I could call upon to become involved with me in parenting my baby and in supporting me. Around Christmas I sent out a holiday letter to a handful of people who care about me, telling them of my plans to adopt. I decided that those people who responded with enthusiasm would be the ones I would invite to become more involved with me as I raised my child. To my delight, the very people I care most about have responded with excitement and enthusiasm as I've proposed how we can make a strong network of love for this baby."

"Imagine my surprise when my parents were the ones to initiate the first conversation about adoption. They said that they knew how caught up we have become in our medical treatments, but that they worry about how focused we have become on a birth child as the only way to begin our family. Both of them know many couples who have adopted, and they were quick to say that some of their children had experienced difficulties growing up. But they reminded us that many families have at least one child who faces problems of one kind or another, and that is a challenge for all parents, not just those who adopt. They reminded us that the doctors seem no closer to diagnosing the cause of our infertility than they were three years ago when we began our workup, and they asked if we had set a time frame for how long we would continue treatment. It really set Matt and me to thinking, since month after month we had only envisioned more medical treatments. My parents encouraged us to open a new chapter in our quest for parenthood, and I'm really glad they did."

"For me adoption was a legal formality that I both welcomed and dreaded. Since my partner and I are lesbians and she is the one who carried our pregnancy, I would not have had any legal rights as a parent unless I formally adopted our baby. I'd be less than honest if I said that the home study was anything other than an intrusion and a reminder that society hasn't figured out how lesbian mothers can coparent without legal intrusions. But it is clear that adoption protects our baby and us in case anything happened to my partner or me."

Surrogacy

Before 1993, when in vitro fertilization (IVF) became widely used, *traditional surrogacy* was the only surrogacy option available to infertile couples who wanted some genetic tie to their baby. For those couples, the woman carrying the fetus provided her eggs and was inseminated with sperm from the donor father. *Gestational surrogacy*, far more common now than traditional surrogacy, occurs when the surrogate mother is carrying a child genetically unrelated to her. In gestational surrogacy, the intended mother or an egg donor provides the eggs, and the intended father or a sperm donor provides the sperm. The resulting fertilized embryos are implanted through a catheter directly into the uterus of the gestational carrier, who has no genetic connection to the fetus.

There are differences in how countries regulate surrogacy. In Canada, the use of commercial surrogacy is banned. However, altruistic surrogacy is permitted, in which a "known surrogate" is involved who does not accept payment for her services. The same is true in Canada when donor eggs are used to attempt a pregnancy; the eggs must come from a "goodwill donor" who is known to the woman with infertility and who will not accept payment for her eggs. In the US, surrogacy is unregulated, and laws vary from state to state. Some states prohibit surrogacy and others require that the intended parents (who often are also the genetic parents) adopt their child after its birth from the gestational carrier. These legal variations by state emphasize the importance of working with a lawyer who is experienced in gestational surrogacy cases.

Surrogates are used in a wide range of circumstances, including when the cause of infertility is the absence, malformation, or inadequate functioning of a uterus; when treatment for cancer has damaged the woman's reproductive organs or eggs; when a pregnancy would threaten the life or health of the prospective mother; when chronic health conditions or necessary medications are incompatible with a pregnancy; when multiple pregnancy losses or IVF failures have occurred; or when premature ovarian failure has occurred.

Although an infertile woman will have ended her medical efforts to become pregnant by the time she decides to use a surrogate, she may still be very involved in *assisted reproductive technologies* (ART) if she decides to donate her eggs to be fertilized (by her partner's sperm or by donor sperm) and to have the resulting embryos transferred to the surrogate. In this circumstance, her involvement in ART is for the purpose of harvesting her eggs, but the focus of attention then shifts to whether or not the surrogate can achieve a healthy pregnancy. The genetic mother may choose to freeze any embryos that are not transferred, or she may donate fresh eggs with each cycle of embryo transfer. As long as the intended mother is donating her eggs, she will experience many of the disruptions, to her life and to her emotions, caused by the careful timing of the ART procedures and the emotional side effects of the hormones she is taking.

Surrogacy is a choice couples make who value genetic ties or who want to have more control than adoption affords. One or both of them may be genetically related to the baby, and they can select a healthy surrogate who they have confidence will seek good prenatal care. In the US, if donor eggs or donor sperm are used, the couple can select the donors. They can select the clinic in which the assisted reproductive efforts are conducted. In concert with a lawyer, the surrogate and the intended parents can agree on the terms of a gestational agreement, which can serve as a guide for ongoing and future behavior and communication. For example, intended parents and their surrogate should decide in advance how they would handle medical issues that can arise, such as amniocentesis, multiple gestation, and potential medical risks to the surrogate or the fetus.

However, with this control come some tradeoffs. Adoption (especially internationally) is somewhat predictable in terms of the time it will take to locate a child. Contracting with a surrogate guarantees neither a pregnancy nor the birth of a healthy baby, and the surrogate may be willing to continue for only a limited number of cycles. The costs of surrogacy are likely to exceed those of adoption; and if donor eggs or donor sperm are used, there is likely to be only minimal information about the donors. As with IVF, there will need to be decisions made regarding how many embryos to implant, how long to store frozen embryos, and what to do with any unused frozen embryos. During her pregnancy, the surrogate has full power to choose how many fetuses to carry to term, who will be involved in the delivery, and what medical interventions are acceptable.

The financial costs of using a surrogate in the US can range between $35,000 and $100,000, depending on the number of IVF cycles required. Costs will include medical expenses, agency costs, legal expenses, and payment to the surrogate (including the surrogate fee, expenses, medical costs not covered by the surrogate's insurance, and travel expenses).

So, just as adoption may be the best choice for many infertile couples, the use of a surrogate may be the best choice for other couples. Here are both the concerns and the anticipations of women who investigated whether gestational surrogacy was a viable option:

"Much as I would like to think of surrogacy as something we could pursue, I just know that we could not afford it if it took more than one or two cycles. It would break my heart to go to all the effort of identifying a compatible surrogate and then not to have enough money to pay for all the expenses involved."

"I've spent months and years of infertility treatments and preg-nancy losses. Since using a surrogate offers no guarantees that we would have a baby after more months of hoping and waiting, I can't see myself choosing such an uncertain option. Frankly, I need something besides loss and grief to fill my days."

"After the chemotherapy for my cancer, my main focus was on getting healthy again. Now that Jon and I are feeling more posi-tive and hopeful about my health, we want to get on with our lives, and that includes thinking about ourselves as parents. The possibility of working with a surrogate appeals to me because at least we could know that Jon would have genetic ties with the baby. After the shock of my cancer, I think that both of us need to have a positive medical experience with pregnancy, and hopefully a surrogate could provide that."

"My mother took DES while she was pregnant with me. As a result, my uterus is malformed and I've been told that I would never carry a pregnancy to term. I've known this ever since I was a young teen, so I've had plenty of time to get used to the idea, and I had always assumed that I would adopt children. But when Stan and I learned that gestational surrogacy would make it possible for us to use my eggs and his sperm to create embryos, it opened up a whole new world. I would be willing to see whether we could become parents with the help of a sur-rogate. And if that doesn't work, then my second choice would be to explore adoption. I'm just relieved that my useless uterus doesn't prevent us from becoming parents."

"We have had two babies born with genetic problems who lived only a few months. I desperately need to have a healthy baby, and it scares me to take the chance of adopting when the birth mother may not have good health, good nutrition, or good prenatal care. With a surrogate, we could be more confident that she would have a healthy baby, although I understand that there never can be any guarantees."

"Chuck and I had just about given up on our hopes for becoming parents when I read an article about surrogacy that sounded really promising. It erased many of my misconceptions and suggested Web sites and articles that I've [since] read. Before thinking seriously about using a surrogate, we spoke to a lawyer so that we could understand what we could do to minimize the risks of an unexpected negative experience with a surrogate. We appreciate how a reputable agency and a good lawyer can improve our chances of working constructively with a surrogate. The lawyer with whom we spoke has developed gestational agreements and helped to educate us on how we could take an active role in the process. He also said that in all of the cases when he worked with surrogates, they were warm and caring women who wanted more than anything to bring happiness into the lives of a couple like us. At this point I think we'd like to give it a try for up to four or five IVF cycles. If no pregnancy results, then we'll need to decide whether to find a new surrogate or to reassess how determined we are to become parents."

"We have a daughter, but I've been unable to get pregnant, in spite of years of infertility treatment. Steve and I have decided that we'd like to work with a surrogate so that our daughter could have a sibling to whom she is genetically related. If it turns out that our embryos don't result in a healthy pregnancy after a couple of cycles, then we would be prepared to use donor eggs with my husband's sperm for another couple of cycles. For us, genetic ties are very important, so if a surrogate isn't the answer, then we'll just accept that the three of us are a family and get on with our lives."

"I was the only adopted child in our family, and I always felt different from my siblings. So now that I'm unable to get pregnant, I'm pretty cautious about the prospect of adopting. I know what it feels like not to be connected genetically to my family. If we could use a surrogate, either with my eggs or donor eggs, at least we could reassure our child that one or both of us is the genetic parent. And we would really mean it when we point out the dimple or the curly hair as belonging to our family! I desperately want our child to feel a sense of truly belonging to us."

Child-free Living

Couples and individuals who have undergone infertility treatment have done so in the hopes of becoming parents some day. When the hopelessness or the expense or the exhaustion of infertility has taken a toll, the next step is to assess how important it is to bring a child into your family. This assessment period is gradual, often beginning during infertility treatment as you desperately wonder when or whether your life will ever get back to "normal," whatever that may be!

The infertility treatment experience has been one in which you and your partner nurtured hopes of parenthood as the ultimate outcome. However, as the months dragged on, as hope began to dim and finances dwindled and life disruptions increased, it also is likely that both of you began to ask how strongly you still felt about your early dreams of becoming parents. Infertility changes people in many ways, and as you reflect on the person you are becoming in the process of grappling with infertility, you may discover that child-free living is an option you are ready to consider. The decision to be child free is distinct from being childless. "Child free" implies an open approach to life that is positive and can lead to fulfillment, whereas "childless" suggests a void. Undoubtedly as you pursued infertility treatments, you thought of yourself as childless, characterized by feelings of emptiness and the yearning to complete your family by having a child.

So how can you envision yourself, after so many months or years of infertility, considering life without a child? Just as the decision to end treatment involves some careful insight into your needs and motivations, so do the decisions about alternatives. Some couples, now well acquainted with the disruptions that medical treatment has caused in their lives, may yearn for an orderly existence once again and may decide that bringing a child into their lives would precipitate more juggling of time, money, career, education, and family relationships. Such couples are understandably exhausted after the tensions of infertility. As they resume their lives without the intrusiveness of medical regimens, they may find pleasures in one another and in other neglected relationships; they may discover that life can be fulfilling even without children. These couples will often make a conscious decision to view themselves as a complete family, to enjoy one another, and to move ahead with plans that have been on hold during the lengthy period of infertility treatment.

In the process of discussing child-free living, partners may disagree on their needs and the impact of the decision on their lives together. As with any decision, both partners deserve time to contemplate new ideas fully and to anticipate the consequences on each of them of a decision to be child free. In many ways, earlier decisions the couple made during their period of infertility treatment allowed them to emphasize their shared goal of parenthood. The decision of child-free living, while liberating at one level, has a feeling of finality to it. If partners differ in their attachment to the goal of parenting, this is a time to consider talking with child-free couples, reading literature on child-free living, and perhaps meeting with a counselor who can help to sort out how important parenting continues to be for at least one partner.

It is not only the couple who will have feelings about the decision to be child free. Prospective grandparents, aunts, and uncles may weigh in, urging the couple not to "give up." These family members may remind you of the huge investment in medical treatment you made to become parents. They may challenge you to direct that same energy to adoption or to considering a surrogate.

The important issue here is that you have the right to make decisions about your future, despite the belief of loved ones that they know what is best for you. Even though they may have been there emotionally for you during the dark days of infertility treatment, this does not mean that they understand the person you have become as a result of this life-changing experience.

So you will need to help them to understand your hope that child-free living can offer its own joys and opportunities for you and your partner. You undoubtedly will remind loved ones that you look forward to having children in your life, even if you are not a parent — the special ties with nieces, nephews, and children of good friends can be mutually very special.

The challenges after ending infertility treatment take many twists and turns as individuals grapple with whether a child-free future could possibly be fulfilling. The women with whom I have spoken have ranged from those who initially cannot imagine a fulfilling life without parenthood to those who ultimately develop a conviction that child-free living is the right choice for them:

"You know, even as we're in the midst of infertility treatment, I find myself wondering what we'll do if I can't become pregnant. For so many years Brad and I have imagined ourselves as parents, yet neither of us is at all interested in pursuing adoption. Frankly, after all the stress and uncertainty of our infertility, I can't see myself opening that same door with a surrogate, even if we could afford the expense, which we can't. So that leaves me asking myself whether I could be happy without a birth child. Heaven knows we have the option of having children in our lives, with all the nieces and nephews in our families. So I find myself asking Brad — on our long walks together or after we've spent a peaceful weekend — whether we ever could think of the two of us as a 'family.'"

"Matt has two teenage children from his first marriage, and he's said all along that he'll support me in my hopes of becoming a parent, even though he doesn't feel that we need a birth child to be a family. That was fine until infertility tests indicated that my chances of becoming pregnant are very slim. So naturally I am willing to explore adoption or surrogacy, and I was completely unprepared for Matt to say to me that he doesn't want to 'parent another woman's baby.' He's right that a big part of my motivation for parenthood is tied up with pregnancy, delivery, and nursing; he's also right that we both have the opportunity to parent his two boys. But I feel betrayed when he says that adoption and surrogacy are options he cannot support. I think we both need to see a counselor because we're making no progress in our discussions, and I just don't know whether I can feel fulfilled in my limited role as a stepmother."

"I actually began to mourn the loss of my dream child during the early days of our infertility treatment. With each failed cycle it seemed more and more clear that I would never become pregnant. I felt a raw agony, a huge emptiness, and an all-consuming sadness. By the time the doctors concluded that they had nothing more to offer, I was seriously depressed. I had refused to consider taking antidepressants while I was trying to get pregnant, in case they might harm my baby. But once I stopped treatment I felt entitled to ask for antidepressants. I am feeling more emotionally steady now, part of which may be thanks to the support of my counselor, part of which is because my hormones are settling down at the same time the antidepressants are kicking in, and part of which is because I've been grieving for over two years. That's a long time to come to terms with all the losses of infertility, and at some level I feel ready to move forward out of the misery I've been in. Chuck tells me that it feels as if I'm finally coming back to him, and I think it's true that I lost myself in the infertility struggle in ways I never would have imagined. We've briefly talked about adoption, but neither of us feels that we have the emotional energy to pursue it. And, frankly, I really want to figure out what is going to make Chuck and me happy as we move ahead with our lives. He is such a sweetheart and even though he never felt strongly about our having a baby, he was there for me every step of the way. At least for now I want to focus on our relationship and how we can rediscover each other and all the non-parenting joys that I know are out there."

"I'm spending a fair amount of time trying to decide whether Mike and I have the strength and the emotional energy to let go of our dream of parenthood and to accept that life without birth children can be good. We know that we're nearing the end of the time when our infertility doctor can hold out any statistical hope for us. Both of us know several families who have had serious adoption problems, and we know we're not interested in pursuing surrogacy. But the real question is, what will life be like for us when we remove parenthood from the equation? We just haven't imagined this before, but we're coming to a time when we need to envision how we can sustain our good relationship and build our lives together without being haunted by the void of an empty nest."

"I'm feeling so empty and lost now that we have ended our treatments. Some of the emptiness is from knowing that I won't ever become pregnant, some of it is from the loss of control I feel in my life, and some of it is from not knowing what the future holds for us if we can't have a birth child. My friends in my support group have been great, but they're mostly still trying to get pregnant or pursuing adoption, and I'm not doing either of those. Bob doesn't seem to be at loose ends as much as I am, probably because he has always said that he'll go in whatever direction will make me happy. But I'm far from happy right now. Several of my support group friends have given me the names of infertile couples who decided not to pursue parenthood, and I think I should talk with them to see how they reached that decision and see how they've been able to shape their lives as a non-parenting couple. And before I ask my doctor for an antidepressant, I think I'll call a counselor that some of my friends say is very sensitive to issues of infertility so that she can help me find some light in this darkness."

"Jason and I often are amazed that our love for one another has grown during this crisis of our infertility. In spite of the stress, in spite of the hormones, in spite of the tears and disruptions and the monthly sadness of my period, we have come to know each other better than we would have if life had been smooth sailing. And through it all, we have said that we have each other no matter what happens. When we ended our treatment a few months ago, neither of us rushed to search the Web or scour the local bookstore for information on adoption or surrogacy. At one level, we just needed some downtime to absorb the realization that a birth child was not going to be possible for us. But at another level, I think we have been more and more comfortable about building our lives together in new ways, now that the shadow of infertility treatment isn't hanging over us. Don't get me wrong — we still think of ourselves as infertile, and I know that a piece of us always will wish that we could have had children. But that isn't going to happen, so now we need to decide how to make new choices about how we can be happy without being parents."

"The uncertainty about why I couldn't get pregnant was our main reason for seeing an infertility specialist. It took a number of months before the diagnosis was clear, and now that I know what we would have to do to try to conceive, I realize that we don't have the financial or emotional resources to go any further. And the more Sam and I talk about it, the more we realize that having children was something we wanted because that's what our friends and siblings were doing. But, as we see them sleep deprived, preoccupied with babies, and barely able to go out with us for dinner or a movie, we've really re-evaluated whether parenthood is what we want. And we've decided it's not. So, in a perverse way, infertility gave us enough time to pause and to decide that children are less important to us than we are to one another."

"We got all the way through infertility treatment with the support of family and friends. But now that we have ended treatment with no hope of becoming pregnant, I'm really feeling stuck. My parents are encouraging us to pursue adoption, but Jim and I just aren't interested in doing that. We've used up so much time and money on infertility that now we just want some time to catch our breath. My sister suggested that it might be useful for us to talk with a counselor about where we'll go from here. She knows me pretty well, and I guess she can see that I am at a crossroads about how to move into the future without the hope of a birth child. Jim says that a counselor might help to get us talking again about what we want, since the focus for so many years has been on getting pregnant. So I guess that's our next step — maybe a counselor will offer some new ways for us to think about our lives together and ways that we can find happiness without children of our own."

"After we discontinued infertility treatment, we first explored adoption. I remember one of the social workers saying that we needed to think of adoption not as second *best*, but as our second *choice* for how to become parents. The more Tom and I talked, the more we became aware that adoption would always be 'second best' for us, and we didn't want to subject an adopted child or ourselves to the feeling of disappointment that adoption was an alternative that we selected out of desperation. So we took some time away from any pursuit of parenthood and tried to think about what could work for us as a second choice. The more months passed without the disruption and uncertainty of infertility treatment, the more we came to realize that we were getting our lives back! Not the lives we had before infertility, but lives where we could enjoy choosing how to spend our time together, choosing new hobbies to pursue, choosing to plan a trip or take a course that wouldn't be interrupted by tests and treatment. What we began to discover was that we were learning to enjoy life as a twosome. That has opened up a whole new conversation about how parenthood is not the only pathway to happiness for us."

"During our years of infertility we found it was very painful to be around friends who were pregnant or parents of infants and toddlers. So we sought out friends who were not parents or whose children were grown and out of the house. What we discovered, even as we were desperately trying for a pregnancy, is that our friends without children were very content with their decision not to pursue parenthood. We also realized from our older friends that their children, while often the source of joy, had also been the source of considerable heartache. These friends helped us to become aware that society tends to paint a rosy picture of parenthood, but rarely shows us the flaws in that picture. There's an assumption that parenthood is the way to become personally fulfilled, but now some of our younger friends are deciding not to become parents, and some of our older friends tell us that they felt worried and preoccupied rather than fulfilled as parents. Once our physicians told us that the statistical odds of our becoming pregnant were slim, we found that we did less grieving than we expected, perhaps because even then we were beginning to realize that parenting has its own sets of worries. Also, we are both feeling very fulfilled in our work and in our relationship, and the thought of adding parenting is different from what it was three years earlier when we began our infertility workup. So now we are moving in the direction of building our lives with no birth children and with few regrets. We've even decided to begin using birth control again as a way of confirming our commitment to being child free. The future looks full of possibilities that we're eager to pursue."

Therapeutic Tips

Most couples have been considering "next steps" before they ultimately decide to end treatment. This gradual process may have been informed by discussion with family, friends, support group members, a therapist, or one's reproductive physician. And, once you decide to pursue another way of thinking about "family," here are some helpful tips to aid you in that process.

Adoption:

- It is important to grieve the losses attached to your earlier hopes for a birth child before moving too far into the adoption process. By resolving these losses, you then have the psychological energy to devote to the process of considering whether adoption would be the right choice for you. It also is important for you to be clear on why you are making the decision to adopt, which will involve both personal and selfish needs. This is the time to discard any savior fantasies of rescuing a child from unfortunate circumstances.

- Make every effort to speak with adoptive parents in your community, as well as attending conferences, accessing Internet Web sites, reading adoption literature, and attending community events for adoptive families. Not only will this give you a sense of the realities of the adoption experience, it also can introduce you to some helpful sources of support as you proceed through the adoption process.

- Your investigations will remind you that there are many routes to adoption, and each one has advantages and disadvantages that you will want to carefully consider.

- Ultimately, you will need to be clear about what kind of relationship, if any, you will want to have with your child's birth parents. You will want to assess your level of comfort with an anonymous, semi-open, or fully open placement. A fully open relationship typically involves ongoing contact among birth parent(s), adoptive parents, and child. The terms of the placement plan need to be clarified before the adoption is finalized.

- Prior to the placement, it will be important to educate and sensitize family and friends about easily misunderstood adoption issues. Share your own literature with them and help them to use correct adoption terminology. For example, the terms *birth* or *biological* parent should be used in place of *real* or *natural* parent; in reference to the termination of the birth mother's parental rights, rather than using the phrases "give up" "surrender," or "give away," it is far preferable to describe the birth mother as "making an adoption plan" for her child. The term *illegitimate* should be replaced by *born to single parents*.

Surrogacy:

The decision to use a gestational carrier often provides the only opportunity for there to be genetic ties between you and/or your partner and your baby. As stated earlier in this chapter, there are both legal and religious constraints that some couples may face in using a surrogate. The costs are generally likely to be more expensive than adoption, so it is important to research all aspects of gestational surrogacy that may apply in your particular circumstances.

The challenges of using a gestational carrier are considerable, and it is important to anticipate concerns in advance, as well as to enlist the assistance of attorneys and mental health professionals to ease your way along this particular path to parenthood. The most common problems fall within two categories:

- Struggles with conception. Simply locating a surrogate is not enough; she will need to surmount the risks facing all pregnant women: miscarriage, high-risk pregnancy, negative prenatal test results, and illness all can occur. Even once there is a successful conception, frequent concerns arise around the difference in perspectives between the carrier, who may feel quite optimistic, and the intended parents, whose history of infertility may have schooled them to be apprehensive and hypervigilant.

- Struggles with the relationship. One area that is likely to present conflict is prenatal and medical care, and the intended parents must communicate early what really matters to them. They also must decide on which issues of disagreement to be flexible and on which to pursue through careful discussion. Even though the disagreements may be about medical treatment, it is important that everyone realizes it is not the role of medical caregivers to mediate these differences — this is the time to engage a mental health professional with skills in conflict mediation and expertise in the particular challenges faced by gestational carriers and intended parents.

Child-free Living:

As with other post-treatment decisions, even during treatment you may gradually have begun to envision a new way of shaping your family. For various reasons, you may have given special attention to the dilemma of what it might be like to revise your perspective from being *childless* to being *child free*. These are healthy growing pains to have, since one of the greatest dangers to remaining childless is in not making a thoughtful and conscious decision to live without raising children. Drifting amid ambivalence can lead to feelings of unfulfillment and lack of resolution.

A more conscious approach can promote personal growth on several levels:

- Just as prospective adoptive parents need to mourn the losses associated with infertility, so do individuals who are considering a child-free future. Painful as it sounds, mourning can also be very therapeutic in helping you to let go of earlier hopes and dreams, changing your focus to new possibilities that can be enriching and challenging. It may be helpful to have some counseling as you do this, since a counselor can provide insightful perspectives for you to consider, as well as validation of you as an emotionally resilient survivor of infertility.

- You and your partner may be reaching your own decisions with different time frames. Keep the lines of communication open, share your struggles and your new hopes as they evolve, and continue to nurture your relationship — remembering how much you both have endured as you faced all the challenges of your shared infertility.

- One aspect of accepting a child-free future is to create and redefine new goals. Doing this can lend a hopefulness to the possibilities you envision for your future, as well as giving you a sense of creativity that may have been lacking during the years you struggled with infertility.

- Even as you may decide to be child free, you also may decide to involve children in your life. Whether through volunteer activities, close relationships with young neighbors or the children of loved ones, or a profession that involves work with children, it is still possible for children to be an integral part of your life.

Adoption, surrogacy, and child-free living are all ways of resolving your incapacity to have a birth child. Yet even when you have reached the important decision about whether or how to become a parent, there is still emotional work to be done.

Infertility will continue to be a part of you no matter what decision you reach. You probably began the infertility journey not even thinking of yourself as infertile. You progressed through medical workups, hope, sadness, confusion, medical interventions, loss of control, hormonal side effects, and relationships with a whole cast of people who ranged from insensitive to empathic. You embarked on a journey that changed forever the person you are. It also probably changed your relationships with your partner and with other loved ones. The person you have become has been shaped by your experience with infertility and the indelible mark it has left on you.

Epilogue:
The Legacy of Infertility

No one endures infertility, with its many losses, and then forgets. Infertility has stolen your trust in your reproductive capacities, tested your trust in medical authorities, and challenged your trust in the strength of important relationships. However, it has also confirmed your trust in yourself, and that you can emerge resiliently from this anguished journey.

But, even as you move forward to face the new challenges that life holds, do not be surprised if infertility is close at hand. I continue to think of myself as having "tucked infertility into my heart." Others view infertility as a traveling companion along life's pathways. Still others, like Barbara Eck Menning, founder of RESOLVE, view it as a friend:

"My infertility resides in my heart as an old friend. I do not hear from it for weeks at a time, and then, a moment, a thought, a baby announcement or some such thing, and I will feel the tug — maybe even be sad or shed a few tears. And I think 'There's my old friend.' It will always be a part of me."[1]

The Aftermath of Infertility

So what are the ways in which infertility is most likely to be felt as you begin your new journey beyond infertility? One is your sexual relationship, which for heterosexual couples has been threatened on several levels. Months or years of timing intercourse to your most fertile time of the month can take a toll on your sexual relationship. You may need to relearn how to move from the emphasis on programmed procreation to the emphasis on sexual spontaneity and pleasure. Another unexpected issue that presents a dilemma is birth control. For infertile couples, the idea of practicing birth control can strike an irrational raw nerve. And yet, for a variety of reasons (perhaps because you are confident in your plans to be child free or maybe because you are readying your home for an adoption or even because you have experienced painful pregnancy losses), an unplanned pregnancy would present its own set of problems. So you, like other couples, decide to practice birth control as a way to end that long period of uncertainty around conception. It represents a way to exert some control over your life in an area that was painfully out of control during the infertility struggle.

Another area that is affected by infertility has to do with how infertility has influenced your thoughts about the number of children you hope to have. Perhaps your infertility has

---

[1] B.E. Menning, *Infertility: A Guide for the Childless Couple.* (Englewood Cliffs, NJ: Prentice Hall, 1977).

caused you or your partner to rethink the size of your family. This can be influenced by the sense of how special each child in your family will be; by the extent of complications during your pregnancy or that of a surrogate; by the ease or complexity of any adoption efforts; by wanting your child to have at least one sibling; and by practical considerations such as your age and your income. In considering these issues, you also may ask yourselves if having more children than you had originally planned is really what you want. (Or could it represent something else, such as the need to prove yourselves reproductively, to protect against the fear of losing a child, to demonstrate your capacities as super parents, or to have repeated reassurance that the pain of infertility need never haunt you again?)

You, like many infertile women, may be surprised at how health-conscious you have become. The focus may be on your reproductive capacities, either because of ongoing concerns or because the initial experience of body betrayal still haunts you. If you have had considerable medical intervention, you may at times see yourself more as a patient than as a person, and it may take time to develop more confidence in your health. Depending on your age, your health, and your energy level, you may worry that you won't be healthy enough or live long enough to offer your children all you hope to give them over a lifetime. Taking life for granted does not come lightly after one has struggled with infertility, and the concern with mortality seems to remain one of the persistent legacies of the infertility experience.

And that preoccupation with mortality extends to your child or children. Perhaps one of the most unspeakable fears that haunt a parent with a history of infertility is the fear of losing the child who is so precious. This sense of psychological vigilance may translate into real-life vigilance about health and safety. On the one hand, you want to ensure your child's health and well-being; on the other hand, you realize that you need to guard against conveying to your child a sense of insecurity or lurking danger. We want our children to be appropriately watchful, but we do not want to make them wary or suspicious in circumstances that do not warrant such feelings.

The Challenges of Living Child Free

Couples who have decided to resolve their infertility by opting for child-free living have unique issues. It is not unusual for one or both partners to question whether living child free was really the "right" decision. This may be even more likely to be an issue if you and your partner have endured disappointments or tensions in other aspects of your lives — work, family, friends, geographical moves, and finances. The hope that child-free living is the "right" decision does not protect you against other life disappointments any more than it does those couples who bring children into their lives.

Living child free does have some built-in challenges, however. One of these challenges is how to field insensitive remarks or questions from people who note the absence of children in your immediate family. You probably encountered these unwelcome intrusions during the period that you were trying to resolve your infertility. But now that you have made the conscious choice to remain child free, you probably have been challenged by other people's assumptions or value judgments about your decision. Particularly insensitive remarks will suggest that you are being selfish to choose a child-free life. Other remarks, intended to be supportive, may sting as well: a friend who offers to trade in all of her children for a European vacation that you are planning;

a relative who complains that her parenting responsibilities have compromised her career success; or a sibling who says, "You really made the right decision. If I had it to do all over again, I'd never have had kids." Supportive as these remarks may have felt to the speaker, to you they may reverberate as a reminder that the option of giving birth was never yours.

Depending on your extended family and the opportunity for your parents or in-laws to become grandparents, you may find yourself confronting the sadness of prospective grandparents at your decision to be child free. Your parents and in-laws who had held out high hopes for enjoying their roles as grandparents may experience their own mourning period as they let go of this life dream. They may convey their disappointment directly by encouraging you to reconsider your options, or they may be indirect as they offer financial support for you to pursue medical treatment, adoption, or surrogacy "a little longer." Adult children, even living quite independent lives from their parents, are nevertheless vulnerable to parental messages of disapproval or disappointment. There is the possibility that such messages can cause a serious rift in the relationship. If you find this rift is troubling and is not resolving itself, you might want to consider asking your parents to visit with your counselor, your clergy, or some other mental health professional who is sensitive to unresolved issues of loss and grief.

Re-evaluating Relationships

Another legacy of infertility is how to continue to relate to the friends you have made during this intense journey. In the early stages you may have distanced yourself from friends who were card-carrying members of The Club. As time elapsed, you probably sorted out which friends were prepared to stand with you through the heartache and sadness of your struggle. And, very likely, you made new friends with other women and couples who were, like you, trying to resolve their own infertility. You know by now that all of these friends relate to you as more than your "infertile self." And in many cases the bonds forged during infertility are enduring and mutual.

One of the most perplexing issues for you as a woman who has resolved her infertility is how to continue to relate to your infertile friends. You still can identify with their emotional pain, even as you have moved beyond that struggle yourself. With each friend the situation is likely to be different. If you have chosen to be child free, your family responsibilities are unlikely to interfere with the friendship, and the absence of children in your immediate family will enable infertile friends to feel emotionally safe when they visit with you at home or in telephone conversations. However, if you are visibly pregnant or have a child in your life, you will need to talk quite directly with your infertile friends to see whether, or in what circumstances, they feel comfortable being in touch with you. You have been there before, so you know how alienating it can be to interact with a friend whose preoccupation with her pregnancy, her child, or with her maternal role is in every conversation. Conversely, during your infertility struggle, you may also have had friends with children who were able to support you emotionally. There is no one answer, but you and your infertile friends need to have a discussion so that the issue is in the open. Ideally you will both acknowledge that you need to be clear with one another about how your resolution of your infertility may present some ongoing challenges to your friendship.

And, if you are a new mother, you now have the potential to become a member of the once scorned Club. You may decide that some of your friends whose pregnancies or parenting roles were too painful to endure can be a part of your life once again. This will depend on many factors, but you very likely will find some of these Club members eager to be supportive of you during your pregnancy or adoption, to offer tips on infant care, and even to provide welcome hand-me-downs.

Your Long Journey

So, here you are, with your life in a very different place than it was when you first began your infertility journey. Certainly you have learned that you are not alone in the feelings of despair and desperation that come and go. These are normal feelings — not indications that you are "going crazy." You also have learned that some burdens may be too heavy to bear alone, or to share only with your partner. If so, hopefully you have found a support group or a counselor who can help you sort out your emotions and your relationships. You know now that infertility is not simply a medical condition. Infertility touches the very core of who you are and causes you to wonder how you will emerge from this unexpected journey. Even in the midst of your efforts to regain some balance in your life, you find yourself making changes and decisions about your future.

Hopefully you have found new traveling companions to replace acquaintances who could not meet your needs. You see the world differently now, sometimes feeling very alone, but hopefully more often feeling grateful for loved ones who try to be supportive. As time passes, you may decide to review chapters in this book that did not feel relevant during your initial reading. Resolving your infertility takes time, patience, and support from loved ones. And ultimately, no matter how you resolve your infertility, it will be an integral piece of the person that you become. The resilience that will come with the resolution of your infertility can heighten your sense of thankfulness; it can increase your insight; it can offer perspective on life's challenges, and it can enhance your sense of maturity and enduring connection with others. Perhaps you are not there yet, but I hope that the voices of the women in this book have offered both practical tips and also an enduring sense of sisterhood with the many others who have undertaken this emotional journey. I would like to join my voice with theirs in wishing you a safe journey and a satisfying resolution.

Resources

ADOPTION, GENERAL

Adoption Council of Canada
211 Bronson Ave
Ottawa ON K1R 6H5
613-235-0344 or 888-ADOPT
Canada
www.adoption.ca
info@adoption.ca

**American Academy of Adoption Attorneys
(members in US and Canada)**
PO Box 33053
Washington DC 20033-0053
781-237-0033
www.adoptionattorneys.org
info@adoptionattorneys.org

American Adoption Congress (AAC)
PO Box 44040
L'Enfant Plaza Station

Washington DC 20026

www.americanadoptioncongress.org

Child Welfare Information Gateway

1250 Maryland Ave. SW, 8th floor

Washington DC 20024

800-394-3466

www.childwelfare.gov

info@childwelfare.gov

Child Welfare League of America

2345 Crystal Dr, Suite 250

Arlington VA 22202

703-412-2400

www.cwla.org

National Council for Adoption (NCFA)

225 North Washington St

Alexandria VA 22314-2561

703-299-6633

www.adoptioncouncil.org

ncfa@adoptioncouncil.org

North American Council on Adoptable Children (NACAC)

970 Raymond Ave, Suite 106

St. Paul MN 55114

651-644-3036

www.nacac.org

info@nacac.org

Post Adoption Center for Education and Research (PACER)

PO Box 31146

Oakland CA 94604-7146

www.pacer-adoption.org

ADOPTION, INTERNATIONAL

Families for Russian & Ukrainian Adoption
PO Box 2944
Merrifield VA 22116
703-560-6184
www.frua.org

Holt International Children's Services
PO Box 2880, 1195 City View
Eugene OR 97402
541-687-2202
www.holtintl.org
info@holtinternational.org

Human Resources and Special Development Canada Intercountry Adoption Services (IAS)
www.hrsdc.gc.ca/eng/community_partnerships/international_adoption/index.shtml

Latin American Parents Association (LAPA)
PO Box 339-340
Brooklyn NY 11234
718-236-8689
www.lapa.com
info@lapa.com

Stars of David International, Inc.
3175 Commercial Ave, Suite 100
Northbrook IL 60062-1915
800-STAR-349
www.starsofdavid.org
info@starsofdavid.org
This network provides adoption information and support for Jewish and interfaith adoptive families.

US Department of State
Intercountry Adoptions, Office of Children's Issues
SA-29
2201 C St NW
Washington DC 20520
202-501-4444 or 888-407-4747
http://adoption.state.gov
AskCI@state.gov

ADOPTION, CHILDREN OF COLOR

Institute for Black Parenting
11222 South LaCienega Blvd, Suites 129, 233 & 470
Inglewood CA 90304
310-693-9959 or 877-367-8858
www.blackparenting.org

Latino Family Institute
1501 West Cameron Ave, Suite 240
West Covina CA 91790
626-472-0123 ext 0 or 800-294-9161 ext 205
www.lfiservices.org

Pact, An Adoption Alliance
4179 Piedmont Ave, Suite 101
Oakland CA 94611
510-243-9460
www.pactadopt.org
info@pactadopt.org

Roots
1007 Virginia Ave, Suite 100
Hapeville, GA 30354
404-209-7077

www.rootsadopt.org
roots@rootsadopt.org

ADOPTION, SPECIAL NEEDS

Family Builders
Oakland Office
401 Grand Ave, Suite 400
Oakland CA 94610
510-272-0204
or
San Francisco Office
3953 24th St #C2
San Francisco CA 94114
415-970-9601
www.familybuilders.org/index.html
kids@familybuilders.org

National Adoption Center
1500 Walnut St, Suite 701
Philadelphia PA 19102
800-TO-ADOPT
www.adopt.org

INFERTILITY

American Fertility Association (AFA)
305 Madison Ave, Suite 449
New York NY 10165
888-917-3777
www.theafa.org
info@theAFA.org

American Society for Reproductive Immunology
830 West End Crt, Suite 400
Vernon Hills IL 60061

847-247-6905

www.theasri.org

info@theasri.org

American Society of Reproductive Medicine

1209 Montgomery Hwy

Birmingham AL 35216-2809

205-978-5000

www.asrm.org

asrm@asrm.org

Canadian Fertility and Andrology Society

1255 University St, Suite 1107

Montreal, QC H3B 3W7

Canada

514-524-9009

www.cfas.ca

info@cfas.ca

Centers for Disease Control

1600 Clifton Rd

Atlanta GA 30333

800-CDC-INFO (800-232-4636)

www.cdc.gov

The centers can provide recent statistics about each fertility clinic's success rates with IVF, GIFT, and ZIFT.

Fertility Weekly Subscriptions

2451 Cumberland Pkwy, Suite 3374

Atlanta GA 30339

888-662-5048

www.fertilityweekly.com

info@fertilityweekly.com

Infertility Awareness Association of Canada (IAAC)
2100 Marlowe Ave, Suite 342
Montreal QC H4A 3L5
Canada
514-484-2891 or 800-263-2929
www.iaac.ca
info@iaac.ca

Infertility Network
160 Pickering St
Toronto ON M4E 3J7
Canada
416-691-3611
www.infertilitynetwork.org
Info@InfertilityNetwork.org

InterNational Council on Infertility Information Dissemination (INCIID)
PO Box 6836
Arlington VA 22206
703-379-9178
www.inciid.org
INCIIDinfo@inciid.org

RESOLVE, Inc: The National Infertility Association
1760 Old Meadow Rd, Suite 500
McLean VA 22102
703-556-7172
www.resolve.org

Society for Assisted Reproductive Technology (SART)
1209 Montgomery Hwy
Birmingham AL 35216-2809
205-978-5000 ext 109

www.sart.org

bdenham-gomez@asrm.org

Society for Reproductive Endocrinology and Infertility (SREI)
1209 Montgomery Hwy
Birmingham AL 35216-2809
205-978-5000
www.socrei.org
asrm@asrm.org

MEDICAL CONDITIONS

American Pregnancy Association
1431 Greenway Dr, Suite 800
Irving TX 75038
972-550-0140
www.americanpregnancy.org

DES Action USA
PO Box 7296
Jupiter FL 33468
800-337-9288 (US and Canada)
www.desaction.org
desact@well.com

Endometriosis Association
International Headquarters Office
8585 North 76th Pl
Milwaukee WI 53223
414-355-2200 or (US) 800-992-3636 or (Canada) 800-426-2363
www.endometriosisassn.org

Multiple Births Canada
PO Box 432
Wasaga Beach ON L9Z 1A4

Canada
866-228-8824
www.multiplebirthscanada.org
office@multiplebirthscanada.org

North American Menopause Society (NAMS)
PO Box 94527
Cleveland OH 44101-4527
440-442-7550
www.menopause.org
info@menopause.org

Polycystic Ovarian Syndrome Association
PO Box 3403
Englewood CO 80111
www.pcosupport.org
info@pcosupport.org

Sidelines National High Risk Pregnancy Support Network
PO Box 1808
Laguna Beach CA 92652
949-497-2265 or 888-447-4754
www.sidelines.org
sidelines@sidelines.org
Provides a network of support for women confined to bed rest during difficult pregnancies.

Turner Syndrome Society of Canada
323 Chapel St
Ottawa ON K1N 7Z2
Canada
800-465-6744
www.turnersyndrome.ca
tssincan@web.net

Turner Syndrome Society of the United States

10960 Millridge North Dr #214A

Houston TX 77070

800-365-9944

www.turner-syndrome-us.org

tssus@turnersyndrome.org

MEDICAL REPRODUCTIVE ORGANIZATIONS

American Association of Sexuality Educators, Counselors and Therapists (AASECT)

PO Box 1960

Ashland VA 23005-1960

804-752-0026

www.aasect.org

aasect@aasect.org

American Board of Medical Specialties (ABMS)

222 North LaSalle St, Suite 1500

Chicago IL 60601

312-436-2600 or ABMS Certification Verification Service 866-ASK-ABMS

www.abms.org

This is an organization of 24 medical specialty boards that will tell you whether a doctor is board certified or board eligible in a particular area.

American College of Obstetricians and Gynecologists (ACOG)

409 12th St SW

Washington DC 20090-6920

202-638-5577

www.acog.org

American Medical Association (AMA)

515 North State St

Chicago IL 60654

800-621-8335

www.ama-assn.org

This Web site enables you to search for information, including educational background, on a physician, based on medical specialty, name, or location. Staff do not respond to e-mails regarding personal medical conditions.

American Urological Association
1000 Corporate Blvd
Linthicum MD 21090
410-689-3700 or 866-746-4282
www.auanet.org

HERS Foundation (Hysterectomy Educational Resources and Services)
422 Bryn Mawr Ave
Bala Cynwyd PA 19004
610-667-7757 or 888-750-4377
www.hersfoundation.com

National Society of Genetic Counselors (NSGC)
401 North Michigan Ave
Chicago IL 60611
312-321-6834
www.nsgc.org
nsgc@nsgc.org

National Women's Health Network
1413 K Street NW, 4th floor
Washington DC 20005
202-682-2640
www.nwhn.org
nwhn@nwhn.org

National Women's Health Resource Center
157 Broad St, Suite 106
Red Bank NJ 07701

877-986-9472

www.healthywomen.org

OBGYN.net

www.obgyn.net/infertility/infertility.asp

OBGYN.net gathers useful information for professionals and patients about different aspects of women's health. The homepage has links to research articles, book reviews, and conferences.

Planned Parenthood Federation of America

1110 Vermont Ave NW, Suite 300

Washington DC 20005

202-973-4800

or

434 West 33rd St

New York NY 10001

212-541-7800

www.plannedparenthood.org

Sexuality Information and Education Council of the United States (SIECUS)

90 John St, Suite 704

New York NY 10038

212-819-9770

www.siecus.org

MENTAL HEALTH

American Psychological Association

750 First St NE

Washington DC 20002-4242

202-336-5500 or 800-374-2721

www.apa.org

Anxiety Disorders Association of America

8730 Georgia Ave, Suite 600

Silver Spring MD 20910

240-485-1001

www.adaa.org

Depression After Delivery, Inc.

91 E Somerset St

Raritan NJ 08869

800-944-4773

www.depressionafterdelivery.com

International Foundation for Research and Education on Depression (iFred)

PO Box 17598

Baltimore MD 21297-1598

410-268-0044

www.ifred.org

info@ifred.org

Postpartum Support International

PO Box 60931

Santa Barbara CA 93160

805-967-7636 or Helpline 800-944-4773

http://postpartum.net

MISCARRIAGE/PREGNANCY LOSS

Alliance for Infant Survival

2701 Burchill Rd N

Fort Worth TX 76105

817-534-0814 ext 2359

www.infantsurvival.org

AMEND (Aiding Mothers and Fathers Experiencing Neonatal Death)
4324 Berrywick Terrace
St. Louis MO 63128
314-487-7582
www.amendgroup.com

Center for Loss in Multiple Birth, Inc. (CLIMB)
PO Box 91377
Anchorage AK 99509
907-222-5321
www.climb-support.org

First Candle/SIDS Alliance
1314 Bedford Ave, Suite 210
Baltimore MD 21208
800-221-7437
www.firstcandle.org
info@firstcandle.org

Infants Remembered in Silence (IRIS)
101 Third St NW
Faribault MN 55021
507-334-4748
www.irisremembers.com
iris@qwestoffice.net

Pregnancy and Infant Loss Center
1415 East Wayzata Blvd, Suite 30
Wayzata MN 55391
612-473-9372

Share Pregnancy and Infant Loss Support, Inc.
402 Jackson St
St. Charles MO 63301

636-947-6164 or 800-821-6819

www.nationalshare.org

share@nationalshare.org

SINGLE AND LESBIAN MOTHERS

AdoptHelp

800-637-7999

www.adopthelp.com/singleparents (for single parents)

www.adopthelp.com/alternativeadoptions (for LGTB parents)

inquiries@adopthelp.com

Family Equality Council

PO Box 206

Boston MA 02133

617-502-8700

www.familyequality.org

National Organization of Single Mothers, Inc.

PO Box 68

Midland NC 28107

www.singlemothers.org

Parents Without Partners

1650 South Dixie Hwy, Suite 402

Boca Raton FL 33432

800-637-7974

www.parentswithoutpartners.org

Partners Task Force for Gay and Lesbian Couples

PO Box 9685

Seattle WA 98109-0685

206-935-1206

www.buddybuddy.com

Single Mothers by Choice
PO Box 1642
New York NY 10028
212-988-0993
www.singlemothersbychoice.com
smc-office@pipeline.com

SURROGACY

Organization of Parents Through Surrogacy (OPTS)
PO Box 611
Gurnee IL 60031
847-782-0224
www.opts.com

Because surrogacy is big business and is unregulated in most states, it is important to do your research carefully. OPTS is a resource for information about surrogacy service providers. It can connect people with families who have used specific providers.

Index